NATIONAL INSTITUTE SOCIAL SERVICES LIBRARY ˙

Volume 33

INTEGRATING SOCIAL WORK METHODS

INTEGRATING SOCIAL WORK METHODS

Edited by
HARRY SPECHT AND ANNE VICKERY

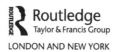

Routledge
Taylor & Francis Group

LONDON AND NEW YORK

First published in 1977 by George Allen & Unwin Ltd

This edition first published in 2022
by Routledge
4 Park Square, Milton Park, Abingdon, Oxon OX14 4RN
605 Third Avenue, New York, NY 10017

Routledge is an imprint of the Taylor & Francis Group, an informa business

© 1977 by Taylor & Francis.

British Library Cataloguing in Publication Data
A catalogue record for this book is available from the British Library

ISBN: 978-1-03-203381-5 (Set)
ISBN: 978-1-00-321681-0 (Set) (ebk)
ISBN: 978-1-03-205803-0 (Volume 33) (hbk)
ISBN: 978-1-03-205805-4 (Volume 33) (pbk)
ISBN: 978-1-00-319924-3 (Volume 33) (ebk)

DOI: 10.4324/9781003199243

Publisher's Note
The publisher has gone to great lengths to ensure the quality of this reprint but points out that some imperfections in the original copies may be apparent.

Disclaimer
The publisher has made every effort to trace copyright holders and would welcome correspondence from those they have been unable to trace.

INTEGRATING SOCIAL WORK METHODS

Edited by

HARRY SPECHT

Professor of Social Welfare
University of California, Berkeley, USA

and

ANNE VICKERY

Senior Lecturer in Social Work
National Institute for Social Work

with

CATHERINE BRISCOE, NANO McCAUGHAN AND CHRIS PAYNE

London
GEORGE ALLEN & UNWIN

Boston   Sydney

GEORGE ALLEN & UNWIN LTD
40 Museum Street, London WC1A 1LU

© George Allen & Unwin (Publishers) Ltd 1977

ISBN 0 04 361025 0 Paper

Printed in Great Britain at the University Press, Cambridge

ACKNOWLEDGEMENTS

We are grateful to a large number of people who made this book possible. First we owe thanks to the United States–United Kingdom Commission for the Fulbright/Hays award that financed Harry Specht's attachment to the National Institute for Social Work as a Senior Fulbright Scholar in 1973–4. Without their programme our collaboration on the subject of integrated methods in social work practice would never have happened.

We are deeply indebted to colleagues at the National Institute. David Jones who provided the original inspiration to prepare a publication on this subject has encouraged us throughout and given us many invaluable comments and suggestions; he also arranged for all secretarial and other assistance. We want to thank Tilda Goldberg and Kay McDougall for reviewing some of the material and for their helpful suggestions. We are especially grateful to the group of Institute colleagues that included Catherine Briscoe, Nano McCaughan, Chris Payne, Kate Griffiths and David Thomas who helped to decide on the outline and content of the book, and gave generously of their time either writing chapters and/or commenting on drafts. The secretaries of the Institute were extremely helpful; and we owe thanks to Diana Broad, Priscilla Foley, Ruby Woodman, Jean Sheldrake, Rosina Shaw and Margaret Theodore. We also owe thanks to the librarian, Maureen Webley, for help in obtaining background material and references.

Peter Leonard (now Professor at Warwick University), head of the Institute's education department, prepared the ground for a book on integrated social work methods. It was because of his belief in the importance of an integrated approach to social work practice that the subject came to be developed within the Institute's curriculum. His successor, Peter Righton, has continued with the provision of support and encouragement during the later stages of our work.

We would also like to thank the contributors to our collection of articles. In particular, we are indebted to Howard Goldstein, Allen Pincus and Anne Minahan. It was strangely fortuitous that their books were published at the time we started our work on this volume; and we are especially pleased that they were willing to contribute chapters to the book.

H.S.
A.V.
1975

CONTENTS

To Daniel and Eliot
and Jason

NOTES ON CONTRIBUTORS

Catherine Briscoe is Senior Lecturer at the University of Singapore. From 1972 to 1975 she was Lecturer in Community Work at the National Institute for Social Work. She trained in social group work and community work in the United States. She has worked in North America as a practitioner and in South Vietnam as a social work teacher.

Neil Gilbert is Associate Professor of Social Welfare at the University of California, Berkeley. His research interests are in the areas of social welfare policy analysis and planning. His publications include *Clients or Constituents*, 1970, and *Dimensions of Social Welfare Policy*, 1974 (with Harry Specht). In 1975 he served as Senior Research Fellow at the UN Research Institute for Social Development.

Howard Goldstein is Professor of Social Work at the Maritime School of Social Work, Dalhousie University, Halifax, Nova Scotia. He has had extensive experience in all forms of direct practice and has served as a consultant to community programmes. His publications include *Social Work Practice: A Unitary Approach*, 1973.

David Jones, OBE, is Principal of the National Institute for Social Work. He has worked at the National Institute since 1962, and was Director of its Southwark Community Project 1968–72. He was formerly Director of the Family Service Units. He was the first Chairman of the Association of Community Workers.

Nano McCaughan is Lecturer in Social Group Work at the National Institute for Social Work where she introduced teaching in group work. She was previously Lecturer in Social Work Methods at the Croydon Technical College. She trained in medical social work, and has worked in the United Kingdom and the United States.

Anne Minahan is Professor of Social Work at the University of Wisconsin, Madison, USA. She has wide experience in social work education and in serving on faculty, agency and professional committees. Her publications include *Social Work Practice: Model and Method*, 1973 (with Allen Pincus).

Catherine Papell is Professor of Social Work at the Adelphi University School of Social Work, Long Island, NY, where she and Beulah Rothman have been involved in the development of the social group work and the foundation practice curricula. Her other publications include 'Teaching the technology of social work: cumulative methods to unitary whole' in Kay Dea (ed.), *New Ways of Teaching Social Work Practice*, 1972.

Chris Payne is Lecturer in Residential Social Work at the National Institute for Social Work. He was formerly Director of an observation and treatment centre for emotionally disturbed children. He has worked in children's homes, approved schools and a centre for adult epileptics.

Allen Pincus is Professor of Social Work at the University of Wisconsin, Madison, USA. He has been a research and programme consultant to the Geriatric Treatment Center, Mendota State Hospital, and has published extensively in the field of the aged. His publications include *Social Work Practice: Model and Method*, 1973 (with Anne Minahan).

Beulah Rothman is Associate Dean and Chairperson of the doctoral programme at the Adelphi University School of Social Work, Long Island, NY, where she and Catherine Papell have been involved in the development of the social group work and foundation practice curricula. Her other publications include 'Curriculum planning for social work education', *Journal of Education for Social Work*, 1974.

Eileen Younghusband, DBE, is now retired. She was formerly with the Department of Social Administration, London School of Economics; and at the National Institute for Social Work. She is Honorary President of the International Association of Schools of Social Work.

INTRODUCTION

'In essentials, the methods and aims of social casework should be the same in every type of service. . . . Some procedures, of course, were peculiar to one group of cases, and some to another, according to the special disability under treatment. But the things that are most needed to be said about casework were the things common to all. The division of social work into departments and specialities was both a convenience and a necessity; fundamental resemblance remained, however.'

Mary Richmond, *Social Diagnosis*, 1917.

'The trend appears to be toward a time when all social workers will need to be able to view the full interventive repertoire of the profession and to understand how the various interventive actions are combined and used in practice. . . . It means that all social workers will be aware of the full range of interventive measures encompassed by their profession, not as skills to be learned but as ways of offering help, influencing situations, and bringing about social change, and will take them into account in their own planning and action.'

Harriet M. Bartlett, *The Common Base of Social Work Practice*, 1970.

Our signal quotations, which appeared five decades apart, indicate that the quest for a unitary approach to the practice of social work has been endemic to the profession throughout its history. Societal changes of the last fifteen years, recent developments in social work practice, new additions to the knowledge base of social work and current re-organisation of the social services have led to an intensified interest in conceptions for integrating methods of practice.

A unitary method of social work practice, to state it briefly, would provide a common set of principles and concepts which *all* social workers could use in dealing with social problems as they are manifest in a single individual, a group or a community. This would, of course, be quite different from present arrangements whereby social workers are trained as, and identify themselves according to, some sub-category of social worker such as case worker, group worker, community worker, residential worker, medical social worker, psychiatric social worker, and so forth. The shift from these specific orientations to a more general one requires a conception of social work functions and goals and of a general set of principles and theories that have sufficient power and force to be useful to a congeries of specialisations, methodologies and functional areas.

Our intention in this volume is to synthesise for teachers, practitioners and students of social work some of the recent thinking that is available regarding these concepts, principles and theories.

The reader who is searching for a definitive statement about social work practice or for *the* unitary approach that is tidy, non-problematic and easy to understand is likely to be frustrated by this volume since that is not its intent. Like all works of synthesis it relies heavily on the work of others, for one of our major objectives is to introduce readers to some of the outstanding material that illuminates the badly lit corridors of principle, proposition, concept and value that practitioners must tread in their pursuit of social work objectives. Also, like other works of synthesis, we attempt to introduce the reader to a wide range of perspectives rather than to explicate a single well-developed point of view. As a result, the reader will frequently find us saying equivocal things like: 'on the one hand . . . this; but on the other hand . . . that'.

Our hope would be that this review of the ideas, issues and problems of developing a unitary method of practice will stimulate the reader to make use of some of these materials in his own work as student, teacher or practitioner. Moreover, we hope that the reader will not accept our synthesis of the works of these other authors as sufficient exposure to their ideas, for that would be an injustice to the reader and to the other authors. Those who are interested in further developing their understanding of an integrated approach to social work practice should become acquainted at first hand with the authors who have done major work in this area.[1]

Several terms have been used to describe the subject matter of this book including 'integrated methods', 'unitary methods', 'the generalist social worker', and 'generic practice'. We have not chosen to use the terms 'generic' or 'generalist'. The former term, 'generic', tends to be associated with casework and was originally introduced to describe the common base of knowledge used in the various functional areas in which casework has been practised (e.g. medical casework, psychiatric casework). The latter term, 'generalist', refers to a particular type of social worker rather than to social work practice. The notion of the 'generalist' as it is used in the Younghusband Report, for example, describes a 'general purpose social worker' carrying a wide range of functions.[2]

'Integrating methods' seems to us to describe what we are in the process of doing as we attempt to find the means by which to join the different bodies of knowledge and the different methods of practice that constitute social work. 'Unitary method' is a useful term to describe what it is hoped will be produced from these efforts. We will use the terms 'integrating methods' and 'the integration of methods' to refer to ongoing work and 'unitary method' to refer to the major objective of the work. We realise that each of these terms is not quite appropriate; on the one hand, 'integrating methods' suggests that the desired outcome would be some amalgam of the existing methods – casework, group work and community work – and this, perhaps, commits us to thinking too narrowly about using what already is. 'Unitary method', on the other hand, possibly promises too much, for the term suggests that the integration or re-synthesis of knowledge and skill has been completed and that the new practice is ready to be launched. Three of the contributors to this book, Howard Goldstein and co-authors Allen Pincus and Anne Minahan, have each written substantial textbooks that describe a unitary approach to social work practice. However, their work as well as the work of other theoreticians in the field will have to be tried and tested by practitioners, teachers and students before it is clear that these are, indeed, conceptualisations of a 'unitary method' that are useful to practitioners, and/or that a unitary approach will necessarily be useful for social work and social welfare. As we noted earlier, our intention is to present the reader with a variety of views and perspectives in order that he may be better able to make use of the available materials and, we hope, test these ideas critically in his own work.

This text is divided into three parts. In Part I we discuss the background against which interests in integrating methods of social work practice have developed and the differences among the models of unified practice presented by different authors.

Part II deals with the nature of the different kinds of methodologies that are to be unified. It consists of a brief collection of relevant papers on this subject that readers will find useful. The collection is small and has been chosen carefully. Our intention was to select only those papers that would help readers to understand the nature of current methodological approaches. Understanding these approaches is required in order to deal with the issues presented in Part I.

Part III is a discussion of the educational and practice problems which we believe must be dealt with as we attempt to integrate social work methods.

Selecting readings for the book was a most difficult task. Notes and references throughout the text attest to the rich and varied literature on the subject matter and readers may wonder why some especially good articles were not included. Apart from the fact that we wanted material of high quality, our choices were guided by three criteria. First, we sought to have contributions from a mixture of practitioners, teachers and theoreticians. Second, we wanted to have materials from the two sides of the Atlantic to demonstrate how the subject matter has been worked on in both the United Kingdom and the United States. Finally, items were chosen to fit our preferred arrangement of topics.

Five of the selections have been written expressly for this volume. We are indebted to these authors for responding so helpfully when we asked them to prepare papers dealing with particular questions and issues. These are the papers by Briscoe, Goldstein, McCaughan, Payne and Pincus/Minahan.

In closing this Introduction it would be appropriate to present the definition of social work practice that we use in our discussion. However, we will not offer such a definition. This is not because there is any paucity of definitions of social work practice.[3] In our view, though, it would pre-empt discussion of our subject matter – which deals with efforts to integrate methods of social work practice – to define a method of practice. We will let some of the authors who have worked on this subject speak for themselves in our review of their efforts in Part I and in their own words in their selections in Parts I, II and III. However, we do begin our work with a particular view about the function of social work in society which, we believe, guides the thinking of many of those who have worked on ideas about integrating social work methods and which certainly has directed our own thinking. In this view, *social functioning* (i.e. the social interaction between the person and his environment) constitutes the major concern of social work. The implications of this notion were clearly stated by Boehm:

'The nature of any problem in the area of social interaction is determined both by the individual's potential capacity for relationships in performance of his social roles and by the social resources he uses to satisfy his needs for self-fulfilment. Hence, the social worker focuses at one and the same time upon the capacity of individuals and groups for effective interaction and upon social resources from the point of view of their contribution to effective social functioning. In the light of this dual focus the social worker initiates . . . steps (i) to increase the effectiveness of individuals' interaction with each other, singly, and in groups; and (ii) to mobilise appropriate social resources by coordinating, changing or creating them anew.'[4]

These ideas have been expanded by others and, by this time, the notion of social functioning as the central concern of social work is well established and reflected in the common use of such terms as 'social functioning', 'social interaction' and 'interface' and 'infrastructure' (the last two of which are used to refer to the social structural connections between individuals and their environment, e.g. family peer group, organisation, institution). Although these words have quickly become part of the vernacular of social work, this view of social work practice requires much more than the coining of new phrases and putting them into the social currency. It calls for the development of a methodology that, at once, takes cognisance of social work concerns with individuals, families, organisations, groups and communities. This is no small order if, at the same time, practice is to be based upon the most valuable parts of the varied fields of knowledge that social workers draw upon and also make use of the skill components that have been developed by years of experience and study in functional areas and in work with special groups and with different kinds of social problems. These requirements for the development of a practice that is based on the social functioning perspective of social work make the task of integrating methods of social work practice a challenging and exciting one.

NOTES AND REFERENCES FOR INTRODUCTION

1 Harriet M. Bartlett, *The Common Base of Social Work Practice* (New York: National Association of Social Workers, 1970); Howard Goldstein, *Social Work Practice: A Unitary Approach* (Columbia, SC: University of South Carolina Press, 1973); Allen Pincus and Anne Minahan, *Social Work Practice: Model and Method* (Itasca, Ill.: Peacock, 1973).
2 *Report of the Working Party on Social Workers in Local Authority Health and Welfare Services* (London: HMSO, 1958), ch. 6.
3 See, for example: Bartlett, *The Common Base*; Werner W. Boehm, 'The nature of social work', *Social Work*, vol. III, no. 2 (April 1958), pp. 10–18; Goldstein, *Social Work Practice*; Pincus and Minahan, *Social Work Practice*; Ruth E. Smalley, *Theory for Social Work Practice* (New York: Columbia University Press, 1967); 'Working definition of social work practice', *Social Work*, vol. III, no. 2 (April 1958), pp. 5–8.
4 Werner W. Boehm, *Objectives of the Social Work Curriculum of the Future* (New York: Council on Social Work Education, 1959), pp. 47–8.

PART I

BACKGROUND TO INTEGRATING
SOCIAL WORK METHODS

In this first part of the book we deal with a variety of subjects that provide an understanding of unitary modes of social work practice. The first chapters develop the background. In Chapter 1 we discuss the societal context of recent developments in social work practice. Chapter 2 deals with the ways in which theory serves as a guide to practice. In Chapter 3 we describe varying perspectives that have been used to bring about a higher degree of integration in social work practice.

In Chapter 4, 'Theory development and the unitary approach to social work practice', Howard Goldstein describes the processes and steps involved in this development. Most important, he conveys a feature of this process that is frequently overlooked, perhaps because it is so difficult to grasp: that is, that the development of theory is a *creative* and a *learning* process. Goldstein provides us with a penetrating and delicate insight into how his own intellectual and experiential perceptions combine to make him a practitioner-scientist.

In the last chapter of Part I, Allen Pincus and Anne Minahan describe their model of a unitary method of social work practice. Their model is based on a distinct view of the nature of social work practice which they describe in terms of its resource systems, functions and purpose. Theirs is an ambitious undertaking. Students and practitioners will appreciate the clarity with which they present their ideas.

PART 1

BACKGROUND TO INTEGRATING SOCIAL WORK METHODS

Chapter 1

SOCIAL TRENDS

Harry Specht

Social trends and intellectual thought of the 1960s encouraged the integration of knowledge in the social sciences and of practice in the helping professions. Several social forces are associated with these trends. One phenomenon of significance was the enormous expansion of knowledge that had taken place in the first half of the twentieth century. The sheer size and bulk of this knowledge made it increasingly unwieldy and difficult to integrate in all disciplines and professions. Social work practice over the last twenty-five years has been enriched by theories about human behaviour (e.g. ego psychology, role theory and behaviour modification), small group theory, theories about community behaviour from sociology, political science and anthropology, organisational theory and social policy analysis. We have only just begun to understand the impact of this inundation of knowledge on both education and practice.[1]

The second major social force – perhaps 'set of social forces' would be a better term – that pushed forward the integration of knowledge and practice is the many-faceted movement for social change in the 1960s with respect to civil rights (of racial and ethnic minority groups, women, students and other population categories that have been deprived and discriminated against), definitions of deviance that stigmatise and disadvantage particular groups (e.g. homosexuals) and political-economic issues such as atomic testing, war, distribution of wealth and consumer protection. In the blazing light of these burning issues the social reform functions which had been historically prominent in the profession appeared to have become pale and anaemic.

And, finally, the social services have become a great social force in themselves because they have grown so large, important and expensive. Social services, which is one of the major items in the national budget of all industrialised countries, has become big business, and social workers are among the managers of that business even though training for the profession has, for the most part, ignored this particular feature of the profession's relationship to social welfare as an institution.

In education, dissatisfaction with, and concern about, the fragmentation of knowledge frequently resulted in the development of inter-disciplinary programmes at an undergraduate and graduate level as well as attempts to make education more 'relevant'. These efforts were manifest usually in more intensive programmes of field studies, in closer relationships between the classroom and the community and in programmes in which students 'learn by doing'. (Some people would view this particular trend as a not very useful one for the development of knowledge and theory for social work because social work and programmes of training for the profession had been, if anything, a too vocationally-oriented enterprise, overly dependent on a narrowly-based, pragmatic practice. From this perspective, social work needs most to increase the theoretical and analytic power of the profession rather than to increase the reliance of its developing professionalism on the field of practice.)

In actual practice in the human services, concerns revolved around fragmentation of service-delivery systems and efforts to achieve better co-ordination of services;[2] it also focused on practice – the behaviour, methods, skills and knowledge of the professional.[3] Social work was by no means the only profession that was subject to critical, often acrimonious, evaluation in that period. Doctors, lawyers, psychologists and other professional groups were frequently called to the public carpet for being over-specialised and (because of their alleged excessive concern with self-aggrandising professional prerogatives) out of touch with the community (especially the poor and the deprived) whose interests they are supposed to serve.[4]

Social work was somewhat more vulnerable to these accusations than other professional groups for several reasons. First, the question of specialisation has been of concern to the social work profession from its beginnings; actually, social work *began* as a collection of specialisations in search of a profession. It was over-specialised before it had developed a basic technology and theoretically-based methodology.

Secondly, social workers work with the poor more than any other group of professionals. Therefore, when the poor were rediscovered in the 1960s and society's consciousness of many other groups that are deprived and discriminated against was heightened, it is not surprising that social work and social services come in for a great deal of critical attention. Indeed, much of the concern and dissatisfaction with social work practice found its expression within the profession itself.[5]

During a period in which human relations and conceptions of human rights were undergoing revolutionary changes, some of the functions of social work that had become fairly well established were bound to be challenged and questioned. Many of the clinical, nurturing, socialising, custodial, therapeutic, and care-taking functions of social workers came to be perceived as means by which society exercised control over oppressed groups.[6] The view of social work as a conservative force was reinforced by the fact that the vast majority of social workers were engaged in carrying out these kinds of functions and relatively few were involved in the social change activities associated with community work, community organisation and social action. Thus, at best, social services were viewed as inadequate, insufficient and fragmented. At worst, they were among society's means for 'blaming the victim' and maintaining an unjust social order.

Studies of the effectiveness of social casework as a means by which to solve social problems further reinforced these views because the findings were, in a nutshell, that professional social casework made *no difference* in efforts to relieve social stress.[7] We do not want to digress from the purpose of this essay to undertake an evaluation of the many evaluations of social casework. However, we cannot pass this subject by without noting that the research design of many of the studies of social casework effectiveness are not well suited to the task: that is, many of the studies[8] deal with client populations who are usually suffering from problems caused by extreme economic deprivation and who did not, themselves, request the kind of help that was proffered by the social caseworkers who treated them. Some studies of the outcomes of social casework interventions have found, for example, that social casework does make a difference in the treatment of people who voluntarily seek therapeutic help.[9] Moreover, in many of the studies of casework effectiveness, the nature of the casework intervention is not clear; in many studies that use control groups it is not clear as to how the stimulus given to the experimental groups (i.e. casework) differed from what was given to a control group. By and large, most of these studies have searched for changes in individual and family functioning brought about as the result of clinically-oriented intervention, a highly unrealistic expectation in the light of the mounting evidence that inter- and intra-personal factors are only one of the many sets of factors that cause these problems.

In bringing questions about the effectiveness of the studies of effectiveness to the reader's attention, we simply want to encourage a degree of scepticism which, we believe, must be applied to all research. Studies of the effectiveness of therapeutic interventions notwithstanding, social work is associated with a vast and growing institution of social welfare that carries out a wide range of functions for the community. The ultimate test of the usefulness of this enterprise will not hinge on the success of any one type of intervention but, rather, on the extent to which the community values the totality of the services performed by social workers. A unitary approach is more likely to provide social workers with a perspective that allows them to plan, implement and evaluate their practice in the context of that totality.

The growth of social work and social services over the past fifteen years has been of a staggering magnitude. In Britain, the recommendations of the Younghusband Report[10] in regard to social work training gave an enormous impetus to the development of social work education and of the profession itself. Estimated outputs from courses that qualified people for social work practice increased dramatically. Figures from the Central Council for Education and Training in Social Work indicate that in 1961 there were 325 people who received some kind of qualification for practice. By 1972, the output increased sixfold with 1,933 qualifications.[11]

An interesting feature of the Younghusband Report is the far-sighted direction it set for the field's growth. Although the field of social work had not yet developed a vocabulary with which to deal with ideas about the service-delivery and inter-organisational problems of which today's social workers are so conscious, Younghusband laid great stress upon preparing professionals who could deal with them. Phrases such as 'combining functions', 'co-operation between workers of many agencies' and 'integration of effort' appear over and over again in the Report.

Social work, the profession, can grow only as rapidly as there is growth in the institutional base that gives it substance and meaning. Thus, growth and change in social work is contingent upon changes in social welfare. Social services have, of course, grown concurrently with, and as rapidly as, social work. From 1963 to 1973 expenditure on the personal social services as a proportion of gross national product rose from 0·3 to 0·8 per cent; and as a proportion of total public expenditure from 0·8 to 1·7 per cent.[12]

The major Seebohm[13] recommendation calling for the creation of a unified social services department in local authorities was given statutory support in the Local Authority Social Services Act of 1970. While the Seebohm Report does not specifically discuss social work practice, its impact on the profession has been quite direct. Seebohm devotes a great deal of attention to the organisation and functions of social services departments. It particularly highlights the social service tasks of prevention, community work and provision of an integrated service. In addition, the Report devotes an entire chapter to questions of the size and needs of social work training.

The clear implication of Seebohm is that social work practice must change. While the forms these changes are to take are not specified, the general directions are perceptible: services provided by social workers should be better integrated than they have been in the past; social services must be able to help individuals deal with their environment which consists of many inter-related parts – family, neighbourhood, agencies, and so forth; social work that relies exclusively on casework methods (whether clinically-oriented or based on practical provision) is insufficient. Thus, in our view, Seebohm calls for a higher degree of integration of social work methods of practice. For this reason, the subject matter of this volume is particularly germane to the social services.

NOTES AND REFERENCES FOR CHAPTER 1

1 See Sheila B. Kamerman *et al.*, 'Knowledge for practice: social science in social work', in Alfred J. Kahn (ed.), *Shaping the New Social Work* (New York: Columbia University Press, 1973).

2 Neil Gilbert, 'Assessing service-delivery methods: some unsettled questions', *Welfare in Review*, vol. XLIII, no. 4 (December 1969), pp. 25–33; William Reid, 'Interagency coordination in delinquency prevention and control', *Social Service Review*, vol. XXXVIII, no. 4 (December 1964).

3 See, for example: Willard C. Richan and Allan R. Mendelsohn, *Social Work: the Unloved Profession* (New York: Franklin Watts, 1973); Richard Cloward and Francis F. Piven, 'Professional bureaucracies: benefit systems as influence systems', in Murray Silberman (ed.), *The Role of Government in Promoting Social Change* (New York: Columbia University School of Social Work, 1966); Matthew Dumont, 'The changing face of professionalism', *Social Policy* (May/June 1972).

4 See Arnold Gurin, 'Education for changing practice', in Kahn (ed), *Shaping the New Social Work*, pp. 169–98; Richard Cloward and Irwin Epstein, 'Private social welfare's disengagement from the poor' and 'The case of family adjustment agencies', in Mayer Zald (ed.), *Social Welfare Institutions* (New York: Wiley, 1965); Gideon Sjoberg *et al.*, 'Bureaucracy and the lower class', *Sociology and Social Research*, vol. L, no. 3 (April 1966).

5 See Richan and Mendelsohn, *Social Work: the Unloved Profession*; Henry Miller, 'Value dilemmas in social casework', *Social Work*, vol. XIII, no. 1 (January 1968); John L. Ehrlich, 'The "turned-on" generation: new anti-establishment action roles', *Social Work*, vol. XVI, no. 4 (October 1971).

6 For an amusing perspective on the social control function of helping professionals, see Kenneth Keniston, 'How community mental health stamped out the riots (1968–78)', *Trans-action*, vol. V, no. 8 (July/August 1968), pp. 21–9.

7 Edward J. Mullen *et al.* (eds.), *Evaluation of Social Intervention* (San Francisco: Jossey-Bass, 1972); Joel Fischer, 'Is casework effective? A review', *Social Work*, vol. XVIII, no. 1 (January 1973), pp. 5–20.

8 See, particularly, Fischer, 'Is casework effective?'

9 Steven Paul Segal, 'Research on the outcome of social work therapeutic intervention: a review of the literature', *Journal of Health and Social Behaviour*, no. 13 (March 1972), pp. 3–17.

10 *Report of the Working Party on Social Workers in the Local Authority Health and Welfare Services*, p. 226.

11 Central Council for Education and Training in Social Work, *Social Work: Setting the Course for Social Work Education* (London: CCETSW, 1973), pp. 26–7.

12 See *Annual Abstract of Statistics, 1974*, Tables 317 and 333.

13 *Report of the Committee on Local Authority and Allied Personal Social Services Series* (London, HMSO 1972).

Chapter 2

THEORY AS A GUIDE TO PRACTICE

Harry Specht

HOW UNITARY METHOD WILL CHANGE SOCIAL WORK PRACTICE

With the development of a unitary method, how will social work practice differ from what social workers presently do? This is a rather simple question and the answer is just as simple: with a unitary method social workers will do the same things that they do now; they will counsel, guide, advocate for and treat their clients; they will work with groups and organisations. Moreover, the thinking that underlies the development of a unitary method does *not* support the notion that every social worker will be expected to undertake every kind of task and function ranging from work with individuals and families to work with community organisations and institutions. Nor does this thinking preclude possibilities of and needs for specialisations in social work practice as both the Goldstein and the Pincus and Minahan texts make clear. Thus, the integration of social work methods will not change many of the features of current social work practice. Nor does it provide any methodology or technique that is not, at present, available. What then, will it do? And why is it important enough to merit our devoting an entire text to discussing what so many people have said about it?

A unitary methodology differs from current practice in two important respects which are best described by the words *choice* and *communication*: that is, a higher degree of integration of the methods of practice will change the way in which social workers make choices about what they do in professional practice whether in diagnosing, treating, or evaluating the effects of their work, and it will change the ways in which they communicate with one another about these choices and about practice. Unitary method, in our view, presents neither a new philosophical outlook for the field nor a new way of intervening. But it will enhance the ability of social workers to make choices that support the field's commitments; further, it will provide a means by which social workers of all varieties can communicate with one another effectively. An understanding of the significance of these features of unitary method requires, first, that one understands how social workers currently make choices and communicate with one another. This understanding comes from an appreciation of how theory directs, guides and illuminates practice.

THEORY AS A GUIDE

Why is it that when confronted with a problem one social worker may decide to offer clinical *treatment*, a second to give practical supports, a third to plan a new programme and a fourth to change the institutional arrangements that impinge on the person(s) in need? One set of factors that affects choice is, of course, the personal characteristics of the worker. This is not an unimportant variable; some workers are more emphatic than others, and some are more impersonal and rational. For example, the increased numbers of males that have entered the profession in recent years will certainly have a significant effect upon the choices made by practitioners since males are more likely to favour rational and instrumental behaviours and females the more nurturing and supporting types of interventions (although, current movements for women's liberation may affect these differences).

In addition, choice is affected by the setting in which the professional is located; this includes both the agency by which he is employed and the professional objectives and behaviours that prevail in that setting. For example, the worker's choices in professional practice in a family service agency are likely to be considerably different from those he would make in a community development project. But to say that agency and setting affects choice is only to say that choices, instead of being made by individual professionals, are made by other, usually larger units, such as boards of directors, 'the administration' and 'the bureaucracy'.

However, the choices we make (even when they are associated with our social/emotional/physical characteristics or with our location in a particular agency) are based on a *theory* or theories. Theory embodies explanations of reality. Whether these explanations are implicit or explicit, and whether they have been tested or not, when we make a choice it is based on some thought that 'x' is related to (or causes) 'y'; for example, that the problem exists because a person lacks sufficient ego-strength, or because the institution responsible for dealing with the problem is inefficient or uncaring. Practice theory is, similarly, an explanation about the expected effects of the worker's intervention: 'if I do "x" the result is likely to be "y" '; 'if I provide emotional support the person will develop greater strength to deal with the problem'; or 'if I get another agency to alter the type of service being provided the person will get more appropriate help'.

A good deal of the theory that practitioners use is not explicit and does not meet the requirements that scientists would set for 'acceptable' theory. Much of it is 'practice wisdom' that has not been rigorously and systematically described, measured and tested. It will always be the case that professional practice will rely heavily on this 'unarticulated' theory or practice wisdom and that is why the professions are frequently referred to as 'arts'. The accomplished professional works with some mixture of well-articulated theory and practice wisdom which is a combination of imagination, intuition and curiosity. In his paper 'Theory development and the unitary approach to practice' (Chapter 4), Howard Goldstein describes how his own practice was given direction by, and gave direction to, theories about practice.

Theory, then, enhances the artistry of practice, and the really creative artist-practitioner builds theory by continually using his experiences to develop new ways of formulating his practice.

A theory, in the scientific sense, is a body of concepts (e.g. 'ego', 'power', 'conflict') that are related to one another by a set of internally consistent propositions. Thus, the following proposition has been formulated by Mayer Zald: 'The more member oriented an organization is, the greater the likelihood of a consensus on action.'[1] The proposition is drawn from a theory that Zald has developed about community organisation agencies. The concepts used in the proposition draw the practitioner's attention to specific features of organisations – degree of member orientedness and degree of consensus; Zald's proposition is a hypothesis about the relationship between these variables. It is a useful proposition for practitioners because it suggests what the consequences of action may be. This is, of course, only one of many related propositions derived from Zald's theory. The important thing to note, though, is that when he uses this theory, the practitioner's attention (or choice) is focused on one set of concepts and not on others. For example, Zald deals with major structural and organisational variables and not with interactional variables such as 'relationship' and 'identity'.

Irving Spergel illustrates how different theories focus attention on very different aspects of a social problem. In 'A multi-dimensional model for social work practice: the youth worker example',[2] he demonstrates how varying social/psychological theories are useful in understanding different features of the phenomenon of juvenile delinquency. The sociocultural perspective draws attention to culturally-induced success goals, social opportunities and the sub-cultural aspects of delinquent behaviour (i.e. the relationships between social and cultural groups and delinquent behaviour); the small group perspective focuses on the relationships among the members of delinquent juvenile groups and the different characteristics of the groups that sustain delinquent behaviour; and the individual perspective provides theoretical approaches to understanding the individual delinquent.

THEORIES AND INTERVENTION

Spergel's article also describes how these different theoretical perspectives lead the practitioner toward different interventive approaches. Thus, he points out how socio-cultural perspectives suggest the development of programmes designed to affect the structure of opportunities for education and jobs; the small group approach leads to intervention efforts with gangs and other teenage groups; and the individual perspective to concerns about aiding the individual delinquent to use available social resources.

From a societal viewpoint it is necessary that all of these theoretical perspectives be employed in order to develop an adequate understanding of and approach to a social problem that is as complex as juvenile delinquency. In any instance, a single perspective will neither fully explain the cause of juvenile delinquency nor provide the basis for designing interventions that will fully eliminate it. For example, opportunity theory does not explain *all* delinquency since much of it occurs among youngsters who are not working class or deprived; moreover, the large proportion of youngsters who are working class and deprived do not become delinquent; nor do programmes based on opportunity theory succeed in dealing with all delinquent youngsters who are working class and deprived. Of course, these same kinds of limitations may be described for each of the other perspectives. The important point is that different theories illuminate different aspects of a phenomenon and, therefore, the wider, more flexible and more varied our theoretical base is, the more possibilities we will have for different types of social work intervention.

We must point out, though, that we are not by any means saying that an enlarged theoretical perspective makes the social worker's choices a *simpler* matter to deal with. In fact, it is quite the reverse; the process of making choices may become more difficult by virtue of an enlarged view. We will discuss the issue of the choice-making process in the final chapter. We raise it here to underline the thought that access to theory determines only the *range* and *number* of choices that are available for the practitioner's use. *How* he makes choices is another question.

Much of the criticism that has been directed at theory as it is used by social work makes the point that casework (because it used an almost exclusively psychologically-based theory) directed most of its attention to the individual's inner life and interpersonal exchanges and relatively little to other variables. This unidimensional theory results in what has come to be called 'blaming the victim'. These limitations of theory as used in social casework have been described in detail by a number of authors.[3] It is important, though, to separate the notion of the validity of a theory (i.e. its *trueness*) from the question of the 'fit' of a theory (i.e. the *appropriateness* of its use in a given case). Freudian theory (and other psychologically-based theories as well) may be quite valid. There is much evidence to support psycho-sexual theories about human development and behaviour. But if its use is over-extended, if it is employed to explain *all* human behaviour, it is being misused; it will not have 'fit'. As Pincus and Minahan put it, 'Any one theory cannot be expected to be adequate for all situations'.[4]

In order to be 'true' and to have 'fit', theories require a great deal of specification about time, place and circumstance. Theories are misapplied when the practitioner loses sight of these specifics. General systems theory, which is the framework underlying unitary methods of practice, may prove to be both a blessing and a curse in this respect: a blessing because it directs the practitioner to take account of a wide range of variables; a curse because he may be spread too thin, theoretically.

As with general systems theory, any of the social and psychological theories we have mentioned may potentially be misused. For example, applying concepts of class struggle to family disfunction or to individual pathology is as inappropriate as applying Freudian theory to an analysis of service-delivery systems.

Poor fit of theories used in practice may occur, we believe, for ideological reasons. Ideologies are single ideas that become social levers, single ideas that are used to explain all social phenomena and to direct all behaviour. Used in this way, any theory such as Freudianism, Marxism, Social Darwinism and Nazism can be turned into an ideology. And ideologies of any sort, while they may be useful in achieving social change (for good *or* for ill), are antithetical to rigorous theoretical analysis. The primary aim of theoretical work is to disaggregate complex realities rather than to reduce them to simplistic ideas, whether to explain inner experience or economic relationships.

ECLECTICISM AS AN ANSWER

The logic of the discussion to this point would indicate that the best practitioner would be a person with a capacity to use a wide range and variety of theories; that is, an 'eclectic'. However, this is not an entirely satisfactory way to deal with these issues for several reasons. First, there are too *many* theories that are relevant to social work and social welfare and it would not be reasonable to expect that all professionals could become competent to deal with all of them. A second and related problem is that many kinds of intervention require practitioners who have been trained 'in depth': that is, some aspects of practice require specialisation in some specific circumscribed knowledge and skill areas and this development strains against eclecticism. Finally, even if all social workers could acquire some working knowledge of a wide range and variety of theories and interventive methods, the problems of communicating the continually developing knowledge and skill would remain. Thus, we believe that while eclecticism, in the sense of openness to a variety of ideas, is healthy to encourage, it does not constitute a solution to all problems of practice.

Before we go any farther in discussion of the theoretical means of achieving the integration of methods in social work, we should like to back-track a bit and consider how the unique development of the profession of social work has contributed to these problems.

THEORY AND THE DEVELOPMENT OF THE PROFESSION

In its origins social work practice stemmed from the efforts to individualise the dispensation of charity. From these efforts social casework evolved. While there are many historical, non-casework threads that have helped shape the profession as it exists today, many of them – the settlements, for example – were related to early social work primarily by their common concern for social welfare. Certainly, in the earlier part of this century when people thought of 'doing' social work, they by and large meant social casework.[5]

Social casework, as Goldstein states, developed without an explication of the 'commitment to and articulation of the philosophical conception of man' that underlies the practice. Goldstein notes that practice of this sort, 'based mainly on a set of pragmatic methods and necessarily incomplete theories is flimsy and subject to change when new approaches come along'.[6] Early social work practice was not theoretically based, and only in the 1920s and 1930s, with the emergence of Freudian and other psychologically-based theories, did social work begin to develop a knowledge base that was distinct from the practice method.

However, social work practice grew in other ways, most particularly with the addition of other practice methods, namely, group work, community organisation, administration and social planning. These other methods differed from social casework in several ways. First, the methods themselves were described in different terms. While caseworkers spoke of 'intake and diagnosis', group workers talked of 'group formation and group goals', and community organisers of 'recruitment and organisational analysis'. Second, while casework was 'invented', so to speak, for and by social work, this was not the case with the newer methods. Group work had its roots in progressive education and community renewal efforts (e.g. settlements and youth work). Community organisation was a creature of the community's organised social welfare interests, political and social action organisations, and university extensions and colonial offices.

And, finally, each of these newer methods had an already-developed knowledge base that was distinctly different from that of social casework. Group work, for example, drew heavily on learning theories such as those developed by John Dewey, on social psychology and group dynamics. The knowledge base of community organisation was fragmentary to begin with but tended to use political science and sociological and organisational theory.

That the addition of new methods was extremely enriching for social work practice is unquestionable; evidence for this can be found in the dazzling array of programmes and services for which social work now provides the primary professional inputs. But this growth and the way in which it has occurred has not been without costs. At an earlier time, 'social work' was what social caseworkers did. Today it includes the many varieties of casework, as well as community work, group work, and administration and planning. One of the major costs of this diffusion of boundaries has been in clarity of communication. Social workers in the different specialisations talk different languages. The milder consequence of our communications problems is to make us wonder whether we all belong to the same profession. The more serious consequence is that we confuse both ourselves and the public in our description of what social workers are, what they do and what they know.

A THEORY TO DESCRIBE WHAT SOCIAL WORKERS DO

The answers to the question 'What do social workers do?' must be cast in a different theoretical framework than that used for any one of the methodological specialisations. It must be a theoretical framework that has 'fit' for the social functioning objectives of social work that we mentioned in the introduction to this essay. The kind of theoretical framework required must be, of necessity, on a higher, more general level than we now use if it is to guide practice choices in dealing with the interaction of the person and the environment. In the following chapter we will describe how social systems theory has been used by several authors to accomplish this task. But in concluding this chapter, we would like to remind the reader of the criteria against which a theoretical approach in social work should be assessed:

(1) it should facilitate communication about the wide-ranging activities of social workers and it should provide a common language so that knowledge and information about practice can accumulate systematically;

(2) the choices that professionals make should be more easily identified;

(3) it should present a body of concepts that are organised in a series of inter-related propositions that can be tested in practice and, thus,

increase the practitioner's ability to predict the outcomes of his efforts; and

(4) these propositions should yield *practice theory* (i.e. directives and guides for action).

In our final chapter we will examine the extent to which some of the current efforts to integrate practice meet these criteria.

NOTES AND REFERENCES FOR CHAPTER 2

1 Mayer Zald, 'Organizations as polities', in Ralph Kramer and Harry Specht (eds), *Readings in Community Organization Practice* (Englewood Cliffs, NJ: Prentice-Hall, 1969), p. 146.

2 Irving Spergel, 'A multi-dimensional model for social work practice: the youth worker example', *Social Service Review*, vol. XXXVI, no. 1 (March 1962), pp. 62–71.

3 See, for example: Sister Mary Paul Janchill, 'Systems concepts in casework theory and practice', *Social Casework*, vol. L, no. 2 (February 1969), pp. 74–82; Ann Hartman, 'But what is social casework?', *Social Casework* (July 1971), pp. 411–19; Anne Vickery, 'A systems approach to social work intervention: its uses for work with individuals and families', *British Journal of Social Work*, vol. IV, no. 4 (Winter 1974), pp. 389–404.

4 Pincus and Minahan, *Social Work Practice*, p. 97.

5 See, for example: Arnold Gurin, 'Social planning and community organization', pp. 1325–6, and Scott Briar, 'Social casework and social group work: historical foundations', pp. 1238–40, in Robert Morris *et al.* (eds), *Encyclopedia of Social Work, Vol. 11* (New York: National Association of Social Workers, 1971).

6 Goldstein, *Social Work Practice*, p. 41.

Chapter 3

SOCIAL WORK PRACTICE: DIVISIONS AND UNIFICATIONS

Anne Vickery

Isaiah Berlin[1] in an essay on Tolstoy's view of history captures the essence of a fundamental difference between individuals who view their multifarious experiences as parts of an all-embracing and intelligible whole, and those whose perception of life cannot be fitted into any kind of single organised conceptual framework. He writes:

'For there exists a great chasm between those, on the one side, who relate everything to a single central vision, one system less or more coherent or articulate, in terms of which they understand, think and feel – a single, universal, organising principle in terms of which alone all that they are and say has significance – and, on the other side, those who pursue many ends, often unrelated and even contradictory, connected, if at all, only in some *de facto* way, for some psychological or physiological cause, related by no moral or aesthetic principle. These last live lives, perform acts and entertain ideas that are centrifugal rather than centripetal. Their thoughts are scattered or diffused, moving on many levels, seizing upon the essence of a vast variety of experiences and objects for what they are in themselves, without consciously or unconsciously seeking to fit them into, or exclude them from, any one unchanging, all-embracing sometimes self-contradictory and incomplete, at times fanatical, unitary inner vision.'

Berlin goes on to say that some individuals, of whom Tolstoy was one, embody this difference within them. They are by nature people who 'know many things' that are different, unrelated and even contradictory. Nevertheless they express a belief in 'one big thing'. Such people carry the burden of having to reconcile what they know through experience and aesthetic analysis with what intellectually and morally they believe to be the case.

A similar burden of uncertainty is carried by social work educators who believe the unification of methodology for practice to be important.

The desire to unify and to find common principles that transcend differences of detail usually does not obviate the fear that important truths may be lost in the process, that the orthodox version of practice could become greatly removed from the reality of the practitioner's experience.

In this chapter we shall examine various ways in which unification has already been conceptualised. Although we do not wish to enter into persuasive argument either for or against any particular view, we nevertheless share with others certain assumptions about the objectives of a unitary social work model and the criteria by which it should be evaluated. The unitary model must be able to accommodate a wide range of approaches and allow for the use of a wide variety of theoretical frames of reference in the assessment of problem situations. It must capture a vision of man in society that is capable of providing a valid understanding of clients and consumers in the context of the social realities of their lives and problems.[2] While meeting the requirement of unification at one level of generalisation it should not result in distortion or loss at another.

SPECIALISED KNOWLEDGE

No discussion of the unification of knowledge for practice is possible without a review of how it has previously been divided. Broadly speaking the divisions were based, first, on specialisation by fields of practice, by which we mean the knowledge required to work with certain categories of clients, usually in a specific kind of agency setting such as a hospital, probation or child care. Second, the divisions are based on specialisation by method, namely, casework, group work and community work. With regard to both kinds of specialisation the position of residential work is ambiguous. While we accept that it is part of social work we do not conceive of it as a separate method. It is easier to think of it as requiring specialisation by field of practice, but this is to raise a variety of issues that are discussed in a later chapter.

Specialisation by Field of Practice

In certain important respects the history of social work education and practice in the United Kingdom is different from that of the United States. Unlike the United States, specialisation by field of practice was especially evident here during the fifties and sixties; and this was partly due to the increase in social workers' statutory functions brought about by post-war legislation. However, there were conflicting trends. In the late forties, child care courses were set up in anticipation of the 1948 Children's Act. Later, in the sixties, following the 1959 Younghusband Report,[3] two-year, non-graduate certificate in social work courses were established. Although generated by the need to train local authority health and welfare workers to implement the 1948 National Assistance Act and the 1959 Mental Health Act, they were taken by workers of all kinds and were in effect generic in their orientation.

Emphasis on fields of practice was partly a response to the way in which statutory functions were organised. The views of some of the influential sectors of the social work profession were divided between those who supported training in special fields and those who supported the 'generic' social work courses or courses in applied social studies which were started in universities in the late 1950s.

A great deal of the history of social work in the United Kingdom between the end of the Second World War and 1970 relates to the struggle between the expansion of specialised fields of practice on the one hand and the drive towards genericism in training on the other.

With regard to this struggle it is important to be clear about the distinction between 'genericism' and 'generalist'. The term 'generic' refers to the common core of knowledge and skills deemed necessary for all social workers in whatever field of practice. As we noted earlier, the term was used largely in reference to different functional varieties of social casework. 'Generalist', in this British context, is a 'general purpose social worker' carrying a wide range of functions.[4] Nevertheless they have become closely associated with each other; and this is probably because the pursuit of a common body of knowledge and skills in different fields of practice becomes less arduous if in fact it is linked with a change in the field that makes the training of 'general purpose social workers' a top priority.

It could be said that the resolution of divergent trends in the field of statutory social service and social work training was brought about by the amalgamation of several of these statutory fields of practice. In Scotland in 1970, the separate specialised local authority departments and the probation service were amalgamated into comprehensive local authority social work departments. In 1971 a similar amalgamation, excluding the probation service, took place in England and Wales, resulting in local authority social services departments. Amalgamation also took place professionally in 1970 with the establishment of the British Association of Social Workers which brought together the separate professional social workers' associations. With the exception of probation this marked the end of the era of specialist workers in terms of fields of practice.

Specialisation in Methods

Many people believe that until recently British social workers have been trained only as caseworkers. This perception requires examination and modification because it refers principally to the era of the fifties and sixties. However, prior to the Second World War social work education in the United Kingdom was largely dependent on university courses in social science and social administration. With few exceptions, training for work with clients was generally done on an apprenticeship basis within agencies.[5] One exception was the mental health course which began in 1929 at the London School of Economics. We will refer again to this course when we come to our chapter on casework.

Here, it is important to note that it did not start out as, and was never intended to be, a specialised course in casework. It aimed, in fact, to give workers who had already studied social administration sufficient knowledge of psychology, psychiatry and psycho-social development to practise with mentally disturbed clients; and it also aimed to inform the practice of workers outside the mental health field such as probation officers and child care workers. The emphasis was not on casework, but rather on acquiring sufficient knowledge and skill not only to help clients and their families but also to promote and support the development of more effective services for the mentally ill and handicapped, and for disturbed children and adolescents. Psychiatric social workers who qualified on this course were involved as much in practice in developing resources in the community as in developing therapeutic relationships with clients and families.[6] Thus, the characteristics of a social work *methods* generalist were more apparent prior to the 1950s than during the fifties and sixties.

Changes that occurred in social work in the United Kingdom after the Second World War were due in large part to the influence of certain significant organisations such as the Tavistock Clinic, and also to American influences. During the fifties, several American social workers were brought to the United Kingdom to give seminars to British fieldwork student supervisers. And many British social workers went to train in the United States and returned to practise and teach in Britain.

Unlike Britain, by the late 1940s, the United States had organised its training in terms of specialisation in methods rather than fields of practice. Students were trained as caseworkers, group workers or community workers. But the cross-fertilisation of British and American workers was mainly in casework. It was, therefore, a method that became very strongly imprinted on British social work education, and the prestige that attached to a practice based on skill in the psychological aspects of casework was too attractive for most workers not to pursue. Inevitably such an exclusive specialisation in one method resulted in an unbalanced view of social work and tended to inhibit caseworkers from using other methods in which they had not been specifically trained, such as group work and community work. Moreover, any form of social work intervention that was not classified as casework was often devalued. These were some of the unintended consequences of the effort to deepen and strengthen the knowledge and skills of British social workers.

The 1947 Carnegie Trust *Report on the Employment and Training of Social Workers*[7] had recommended that the syllabus in 'principles and practice of social work' in new courses deal with 'both the principles and practice common to all forms of casework and group work and should be taken by all students'. Despite this recommendation, the applied social studies courses that developed as a result of this Report continued from 1958 until comparatively recently to concentrate on casework and to exclude group work almost entirely. Social work practice was still conceived as a collection of specialisations with 'field of practice' as the main specialist dimension, with casework as the core social work method. Insofar as there was a common knowledge base or 'generic' content to all these training courses, it rested in the casework method and, broadly speaking, in those aspects of psychology, sociology, medicine, ethics, law, applied economics and social administration that all caseworkers would be required to understand.

Despite the concentration on casework as *the* method of professional social work, other methods were being used as well, both by professionally qualified social workers, and by group and community workers and social service administrators. These workers were qualified in other ways than through professional social work. The development of group work and community work in this country is described in Chapters 9, 10 and 11. The important point to be made for the moment is that, historically, British social work was never confined to casework, even during the fifties and sixties. However, for various reasons the professional recognition of group work and community work as areas of social work education has been long delayed. The profession has been fragmented in terms of methods specialisations, and its knowledge and skill are incomplete and unevenly developed. Specialisation by method has never officially happened.

THE SEARCH FOR UNITY

The search for a unifying framework has taken a different form in the United States than in the United Kingdom. Whereas in the last two decades we have sought to unify specialised caseworkers in one professional body, to provide a common social work education and to unify administratively most of our statutory social services, the Americans in varying degrees have been concerned with conceptualising the whole of social work practice in a unitary method. The purpose of this unification is not only to bring casework, group work and community work under one roof but, perhaps more importantly, to avoid fragmentation and distortion in the reality of people's lives.

In the same way that the British social worker is concerned to avoid defining client problems solely in terms of his or her agency's function, the American social worker is concerned to avoid defining problems exclusively in terms of his or her particular method of practice. Although this latter concern is shared by British social workers, it is perhaps overshadowed by concern that our development in work with groups and communities lags behind our development in work with individuals and families.

The Effect of Social Services Departments
The unification of local authority services has given the British social worker extensive responsibility to deal with a wide range of problems. Sometimes this wide range resides within one family: for example, one family may have a child care problem, a mental health problem and the problem of an ageing bedridden person. One of the main preoccupations of the Seebohm Committee was to ensure that unless there were professional contra-indications, one worker would deal with all of the problems of the one family.[8] Legally, the local authority social worker may now act on this expectation of comprehensive service giving; but it may still be limited in effectiveness because of limited conceptual and methodological ability to move outside a circumscribed area in work with individuals and families. For example, the problems of the one family might be partly due to serious housing difficulties that are endemic to the neighbourhood, or partly due to general social isolation in a new housing estate. If so, lack of a method to make an impact on these wider environmental problems may seriously impair the outcome of the worker's efforts.

A recurring theme of the Seebohm Report is the need to make available a more varied response to client problems. The Committee was alert to the need to broaden the range of social work intervention in the new local authority departments. It said that an effective family service must be concerned with the prevention of social distress. General prevention was defined as the creation of environments conducive to social well-being by improving work opportunities and conditions and by ensuring reasonable standards of living and educational attainment.[9]

'Genericism' in Methods
At the same time that social workers were unifying professionally and local authority personal social services were unifying administratively, group work, community work and residential social work were being recognised, albeit reluctantly in some quarters, as part of social work. Although not all group workers and community workers see themselves as social workers (nor is it appropriate that they all should), the requirements of intervention on a broad front have forced social work education to grapple with group work and community work as well as with casework.

It is important that trainers be clear about the choices open to them as they begin to incorporate this additional knowledge into training for the profession. One option is to absorb some existing courses in group work and community work and also to promote new ones. But this would promote specialisation by method and exacerbate the fragmentation that the Americans are trying to overcome. Another option is to search for the generic knowledge and skills that workers in all of the methods need to have and to build courses around that generic core. This latter option is the one that has led to unitary conceptualisations of practice, and the one that this book is about.

Before describing these unitary conceptualisations, we should review briefly some of the alternative designs that have been developed to bring about unification of practice.

Social Work as a 'Continuum' of Methods

The Seebohm Committee strongly emphasised the need for forms of intervention in the social worker's repertoire to supplement casework approaches, and it wanted to extend the concept of generic training to include the idea of equipping students 'to work as appropriate with individuals, groups and communities'. The Report states that:

> 'The justification for this approach is the belief that the different divisions between methods of social work are as artificial as the difference between various forms of casework and that in his daily work the social worker needs all these methods to enable him to respond appropriately to social problems which involve individual, family, group and community aspects. This newer concept of generic training has obvious attractions as a preparation for work in the social service departments.'[10]

The Committee recognised that the present length of training in this country would not allow for skill development in more than one method. It suggested that although future basic training courses would require all students to study one method in depth, students would learn the generic aspects of all social work methods. In doing so they would not only gain knowledge of methods other than the one in which they chose to specialise but would develop also an understanding of the inter-relatedness of methods.

Although teaching about group and community work is now included in basic training, students continue to concentrate mostly on casework. The notion of a generic content that might unify the trinity of casework, group work and community work method seems partially to have been lost, and the view of the Younghusband Report suggesting the need for separate training in group and community work seems largely to have prevailed.[11] However, the view does not carry the intention to divide and fragment. Rather, it is believed that additional courses will extend the range of skill and understanding of the individual worker who moves along a kind of continuum from casework through group work to community work.

With this view, group work is explicitly seen as the unifier of the two ends of this continuum. The argument for group work as the unifier rests on the need for different types of social workers (e.g. residential social workers, caseworkers with family groups, community workers in community groups and inter-group situations) to have a sound knowledge of group dynamics and the skill to handle them. That is, all social workers working in agencies and on worker teams, and not just group workers, require this knowledge. Eileen Younghusband[12] explicitly takes this view. She also raises the problem of the antipathy towards social work in general and casework in particular that is currently expressed by some community workers. She presents, but leaves unresolved, the issue of how different objectives may affect group work practice. For example, is the use of group dynamics in therapeutic groups different from its use in the inter-group situations of community work?

The objectives of different practices (like social group work and community work) are, of course, related to values. While there are those who believe that there is inherent conflict between the values of caseworkers and community workers, we think the true state of affairs is more complex than this polarisation suggests. It seems likely that there are as many value conflicts between workers practising the same method as there are between different methods workers. It would be important to explore this before abandoning the notion that there is sufficient 'genericism' between the methods to act as a unifying force.

Partial Integration: Social Work Divided Between Direct-Service and Indirect Services

'Direct work' is often contrasted with 'indirect work'. But these terms are often used with different meanings.

Frequently the terms 'direct' and 'indirect' refer to the distinction between intervention in which the practitioner relates to the identified client or client group ('direct') and intervention in which the practitioner on the client's behalf relates to individuals, groups and agencies in the client's environment ('indirect').[13]

The latter intervention is designed to influence the client's behaviour and/or circumstances by indirect rather than direct means. A narrower use of 'direct' and 'indirect' is made by Vinter[14] examining specific types of worker intervention in groups. He refers to attempts on the part of the worker to influence an individual in the group by relating to him personally as 'direct', and to attempts to influence an individual through intervention in the structural relations of the rest of the group as 'indirect'. Vinter uses the term 'extra-treatment' for work that either symbolically or concretely relates to the external world outside the immediate group setting.

A further meaning that might be given to 'direct' and 'indirect' relates to the existential experience of the worker. 'Direct' work, here, involves the worker directly in the problem situation itself, for example, influencing parents to deal in a certain way with their child's problematic behaviour by being present and controlling the parents' activities at the moment the child's problematic behaviour occurs.[15] More obvious examples of this meaning of 'direct' arise in residential therapeutic work, particularly with children and adolescents, in unattached youth work, in some types of work with drug abusers and vagrants, and in the type of work that the early family service units did with families suffering multiple deprivations.[16] 'Indirect' work involves discussion with the individual or group about problematic situations, behaviours and relationships without the worker ever being present in the context in which these problems occur.

These various distinctions between 'direct' and 'indirect' work are useful ones for the individual practitioner concerned with methodological choice in work with clients. None of them has ever been considered the basis for division of labour between different kinds of worker; but broader meanings of 'direct' and 'indirect' have. Under these broader headings 'direct' work refers to encounters with clients (i.e. individuals, families and groups) and includes also all of the work on their behalf with other agencies, professionals and other members of the community. 'Indirect' work refers to activities concerned with the development and allocation of social service resources, inter-organisational work, policy formulation and change, and social planning. It clearly includes major aspects of community work.

Gilbert and Specht[17] give the terms this broader meaning. While wishing to avoid having separate kinds of training, they nevertheless argue the case for distinctively different training for the two kinds of worker. Another writer who uses the terms 'social intervention' and 'societal intervention' synonymously with Gilbert and Specht's 'direct' and 'indirect' is Werner Boehm, who says:

> 'Two types of social work practitioners are needed today and tomorrow: one who is skilled in helping individuals, families and small groups to deal with and change troublesome situations in which they find themselves, and another who is skilled in the strategies of social change.[18]

The division between workers who, on the one hand, work mainly face-to-face with clients and consumer groups and with others on their behalf, and workers who, on the other hand, are concerned with resource provision, policy change and prevention has a long academic tradition in this country. Professional social work has been viewed as the concern of the first, and the academic discipline of social administration as the concern of the second. However, in practice the division is not clear. This lack of clarity is obviously felt by Boehm. He suggests that case-work and group work may not be sufficient for the kind of direct work he has in mind, and that traditional community organisation may be insufficient for indirect work. In the same article he speculates about a new method that may have its own unique identity rather than a bor-rowed one. Here, Boehm may have been anticipating the need for unitary conceptualisations.

For the United Kingdom it is important to note the role that social administration has played in the education of social workers. Tradition-ally, social administration has been concerned with teaching about the structure and function of social services, and social policy and legisla-tion, either as an attenuated subject in a two-year professional social work course or as a complete course taken prior to professional training. It has been a somewhat ill-defined subject and until recently has not been addressed to the practical procedures required to effect the best possible links between controllers of resources, service providers and consumers.[19] It in fact informs and illuminates the work of both direct and indirect workers, but is not sufficient in itself for either kind of practice. Despite this, many professionally trained social workers, as they are promoted to managerial positions in social service agencies, enter into 'indirect' work. In doing so they become engaged in many, if not all of the activities that come under the American heading of 'com-munity organisation' and under the British heading of 'community work', which includes inter-organisational work and social planning. There is consequently a growing tendency for social workers to feel the need for training in indirect work (sometimes called 'social service management' and sometimes 'community work'). Many would see this training as an extension of professional social work rather than as some-thing more closely allied to 'social administration'. Again, this reflects a 'continuum' view

Those who would support the direct/indirect division have to clarify the position of community work. Sometimes, the way in which it is defined and practised leaves ambiguous the question of its position within the 'indirect'/'direct' dichotomy. For example, the Gulbenkian Report[20] on training for community workers identifies three strands in community work: (1) direct work with local people for the purpose of helping them define and achieve their goals; (2) inter-organisational work to bring services and needs in closer relation; and (3) community plan-ning and policy formulation. The second and third strands clearly denote indirect intervention, but the first is clearly direct. In actual practice, though, practitioners in community development or 'grass roots' community work vary in the emphasis they give to either side of the direct/indirect dichotomy. For some, the emphasis is on what the community groups set out to achieve, such as additional resources, changes in agency policies, the creation of new amenities, and an increase in social cohesion and mutual support. All these aims are consonant with a definition of indirect work. Other practitioners, however, emphasise the social learning and personal growth of individuals and groups involved in community work. Despite the expressed goals of community groups, the second emphasis on grass roots community work is close to the direct work of social group work, particularly the 'social goals' model described by Rothman and Papell.[21] Discussing this difficulty in definition, David Jones writes:

'. . . community development comes very close to group work . . . in fact one might see the activities discussed hitherto as a continuum consisting of casework/group work/community development/community organisation/social administration. While no clear-cut distinction is possible or desirable, the primary emphasis on the casework/group work end of the continuum is on individual and group development, while on the other it is on collective action in relation to the environment or community. We shall, therefore, use the term "community work" to cover the broad range of activity on the far end of the continuum which includes work with community groups, administration and social planning.

'An important distinction among these activities can be made in terms of the "client". In casework and group work this is relatively clear. With community development the situation becomes more complicated, for the people involved are explicitly or implicitly representative of a wider group, some of whom in fact may be in opposition to the proposal.'[22]

In this view, the structural relations of the group within a wider social context will help to identify whether the work is direct or indirect. However, many who use the term 'indirect services' do not believe that it includes 'grass roots' work or community development. This is clearly one of the problems of the direct/indirect division of labour.

There is a further difficulty that will become evident later on when we discuss the importance of the exchanges among individuals and between people and social institutions as the major focus of social work. Unless the 'linkages'[23] between the education of direct-service and of indirect-service workers are very well managed there is the risk of impoverishment in social work practice. Hartman writes:

'Such a dichotomous view, although including the poles of the continuum, tends to create two different professions and to exclude the middle range of practice which is focused on the inter-face between client systems and social institutions, a range which includes, among others, developmental, social broker, mediation, and case advocacy roles – a range which many would define as the heart of social work practice.'[24]

Middleman and Goldberg.[25] in their conceptualisation of micro-level social work practice, overcome this dichotomy by making work with community groups the province of both the direct-service worker and the indirect-service worker. In common with others, these authors use the words micro-level intervention and macro-level intervention to denote, respectively, direct and indirect work; and they suggest that intervention with resource holders on behalf of individual clients (clearly the province of the micro-level worker) may at times become the province also of the macro-level worker. In effect they outline a unitary conceptualisation of social work practice that delineates the boundaries of both the direct and indirect-service worker so as to provide substantial areas of overlap. In developing their text they intentionally confine themselves to the work of the direct-service worker. But the text is conceived within a unitary framework.

By contrast, Whittaker places work with community groups into the macro-level area of practice.[26] Although, like Middleman and Goldberg, he confines the details of his text to the knowledge and skills required of a micro-level practitioner, his conception of micro-level practice is very different. Besides the common social work process of planned change, his unifying ingredients consist mainly of the various theories and forms of social treatment that are equally applicable in work with individuals, families and groups. He does not discuss how the dichotomy between the micro- and the macro-level worker might be bridged.

A major part of the difference between the texts of Middleman/Goldberg and Whittaker stems from the differing views of the authors about the aims of social work. Whittaker clearly believes that social work is to do both with helping people directly in their social functioning and with changing institutions. Middleman and Goldberg take up a value position that confines the aims of social work to structural change. As we shall see, a more narrowly focused definition of the problem makes the unification of social work practice much easier.

The 'Problem' as the Unifier
So far we have been considering the extension of knowledge and skill in 'methods'. We have delineated, on the one hand, the 'continuum' view

regarding unity and, on the other, the view that the former divisions of casework, group work and community work should be replaced by a new division between direct-service and indirect-service work. However, there are those who question the validity of a 'methods' orientation, whether viewed as a continuum or as direct/indirect. Without underestimating the importance of skill development, they place the *nature of the human problem* and the *purpose* of the work to be done in the foreground, and they relegate the technology of doing it to a less important position. In so doing they emphasise the need to organise knowledge around the particular human problem on which the social worker is required to have an impact such as the social problems of disadvantaged children, or the aged or the handicapped. Maas argues that technology should be studied and applied only in relation to a target population.[27] He writes: 'Social work students can no longer be educated to help mankind – except in the most superficial and therefore professionally irresponsible ways.'[28] In his view, social work must make use of the specialist knowledge that has burgeoned in many areas of human life and interaction. It should not be ignored for the sake of developing a detailed but narrow conception of human problems limited by the range of the one social work method in which the practitioner is specialised. Nor should social work develop a global conception of human problems that fails to provide sufficient boundaries and specificity for appropriate and responsible action.

This latter danger is also the concern of Gilbert and Specht in their identification of the basic differences in the academic requirements and practice orientations of direct-service and indirect-service practitioners. In their view, courses that prepare students for both kinds of service and that require that all students take the same subjects 'tend to emphasise the objective of professional unity at the cost of functional relevance'.[29] Maas, however, like Hartman, has misgivings about a 'two-track' format for social work education based on the direct/indirect service dichotomy, and emphasises the inseparability of the human problem into different methods. He says:

'The one-to-one worker who is also at times advocate and mediator and policy developer and implementer will be unable to win the trust of the so-called indirect-service community worker – whose work is actually *directly* with some of the same people more often than the unfortunate *indirect* service label suggests. In graduate school, students preparing for work with black communities or in community health programmes will see, time and again, that the complexities of the problems with which one worker deals *demand* the collaborative efforts of another worker entering the problem situation at another level, with a different kind of intervention. . . .'

'The artificial divisions of underlying academic disciplines provide no rational bases for the segmentation of professional education, purpose and practice.'[30]

While addressed to the same issue of delineating professional activities so that students acquire relevant knowledge and practice orientations, Maas advocates an entirely different dimension for delimitation than the direct/indirect. Partly, he is concerned that social work education should not be divided in such a way as to impair working relationships between social work specialists and non-social work professionals. But his primary concern is probably less with this issue and more with the need for adequate knowledge from a wide variety of sources to be available to all the practitioners involved in work on a particular problem.

Although Maas relegates methodological issues to the background, his demands of social work practice require that it be conceptualised as a unitary activity.

The case of 'The House on Sixth Street'[31] is a nice illustration. Here a team of social workers which included caseworkers and group workers focused their efforts on the problems of the tenants of a slum dwelling. These tenants had many problems requiring individualised help. But they held in common the problems attendant on living in a rat-infested building lacking gas, electricity and hot water, and in which homeless men and addicts were squatting. The case exemplifies a generalist approach in terms of the methods of intervention, but a specialist approach in terms of problem focus – in this instance, housing. The workers sought to bring about change in several interacting social systems in which the problem of the particular tenement block was located, such as service agencies, public utilities and the legal system. They also supported and sustained individual tenants and families and enabled them to negotiate with various agencies and to organise themselves into a pressure group. There was practically no differentiation of task between the two principal workers, one of whom was trained in community organisation. They drew in caseworkers who 'were especially helpful in dealing with some of the knotty and highly technical problems connected with public agencies'; and also a lawyer and a city planner. Purcell and Specht comment: 'Social work helping methods are so inextricably interwoven in practice that it no longer seems valid to think of a generic practice as consisting of casework, group work, or community organisation skills as the nature of the problem demands.' They also comment on the need for specialised knowledge of the problem in a wide context: 'Although the needs of the client system enable the agency to define its goals, the points and methods of intervention cannot be selected properly without an awareness and substantial knowledge of the social systems within which the problem is rooted.'

In this country the impact of the local authority social services re-organisation and the partial ending of specialised training in fields of practice has tended to diminish an emphasis on the need for special knowledge in particular problem areas. Vickery[82] writing approximately one year after the setting up of the local authority social services departments raises certain issues about the non-availability of specialised knowledge resulting from the generalist approach and the rapid promotion of the most skilled and knowledgeable workers.

It was already evident even in 1972 that lack of sufficient knowledge of particular problems at fieldwork level was influencing departments that had 'gone generic', to backtrack by encouraging the return of certain forms of specialisation, however modestly defined. Even so, for various reasons social services departments are, generally, far from ready to offer the range of problem-focused interventions that Maas envisages, and 'The House on Sixth Street' illustrates. And, for partly different reasons, it is equally difficult for other types of social service agencies to organise simultaneous interventions at several levels of a problem. Exceptions to this may be found in the work of problem-focused agencies like the family service units. Increasingly these agencies use group and community work as well as casework.[83] Consortia of agencies are often able to bring a very rich body of knowledge, skills and resources to bear on a single problem. The Camberwell Council on Alcoholism is an example of an agency which involves the pooling of medical, educational and social work knowledge and the co-ordination of counselling, psychiatric, day-care and residential services.[84]

It is agencies like these, and records of practice like 'The House on Sixth Street', that have enabled unitary conceptualisations of social work to approximate more closely to the realities of good practice, and to overcome unhelpful divisions between methods specialists.

A UNITARY APPROACH: GENERICISM IN METHOD

To state that it is the problem-focus that should be the unifier is to suggest a return to specialisation by 'field of practice'. However, the way in which fields of practice are now conceptualised has changed since the days of specialisation in Britain in the fifties and early sixties. Despite the uneven development of methods, understanding of the contribution of group work and community work has increased considerably in the last decade. This understanding has provided new insights into how some of our more intractable problems might be more effectively tackled if intervention were undertaken concurrently in the various levels in which the problem is embedded; that is, if problems were dealt with at individual, family, group, organisational and community levels.

Social Systems Theory

These insights have also been assisted by the growing number of writers who advocate the use of a social systems perspective on social problems.[35] These writers select aspects of general systems theory that are especially useful to social work. It is possible here to mention briefly only a few. However, the feature of the systems approach which for our discussion has over-riding importance is its capacity to provide a unifying framework for the whole of social work practice. Several authors, notably Pincus and Minahan[36] and Goldstein[37] have recently formulated unified models of practice. All of them aim to incorporate casework, group work and community work within the one model; and all are dependent on social systems theory for a framework in which the model is embedded. Pincus and Minahan's use of a systems approach is implicit, while Goldstein's is explicit.

Social Systems Framework. Social systems theory orders social phenomena at various levels of complexity: (1) the individual personality system which is an intra-personal psycho-biological system; (2) the social system of the dyad; that is, two inter-relating people who form an interpersonal system; (3) slightly larger interpersonal social systems of small groups which include natural groups like the family as well as groups formed for particular purposes; and (4) larger social systems such as organisations, communities and societies that can be analysed only from a socio-cultural standpoint. Any one of these systems is itself composed of sub-systems and is, at the same time, part of some larger system.

Permeable Boundaries. Social systems theory assumes that each system is open to exchange from, and influence by, other systems in its environment. And it further assumes that the behaviour of any one system is understandable chiefly in relation to its interaction with others. This has the effect of focusing social work attention on the relationships *between* systems rather than on the internal functioning of any one system. For example, in helping a family, the social worker will not only work with the relationships among family members, but also with the relationships between the family and relevant service agencies.

Equifinality. A further consequence of the assumed ability of one system to influence another is that it makes one question the notion that problems experienced at any one level of systemic organisation must necessarily be dealt with at that level. It is, rather, assumed that change in any one system has the potential to influence others to which it is relating. Given the multifaceted exchanges in which most systems engage it is possible to believe that a change toward a particular 'end state' can

be brought about by a variety of means. No one method or one level of
intervention is, necessarily, uniquely suited to bring about the desired
change. This has obvious implications for social workers, not only
because it frees the mind to seek for alternative systems in which change
might be feasible, but also because it forces the social worker to consider the relative strengths of a variety of systems by which the client
system is influenced. Vickery's case of Mrs X illustrates these considerations.[38] Here, Mrs X, suffering from depression, is referred by her
psychiatrist for social work help because of difficulties in managing her
children. She lives in a dreary unfriendly housing estate far from her
family of origin. In trying to help her, various alternatives are open:
greater attention and more understanding on the part of the psychiatrist; more effective medication; providing a home help to ease the strain
of being a housewife; work with the children, or with her husband, or
with the whole family to alter family role relationships; group work
with the children and other children in the neighbourhood; work with
the tenants of the estate to decide how to improve their conditions; work
with service organisations to improve service delivery; and so on.
Assuming that no one system is stronger than the other in holding the
present state of Family X in being, the first questions in planning intervention are to do with the feasibility of change. Where is it likely that
change can be effected? Who would be willing to work toward change?
Who would allow change to occur? Once what is feasible has been
assessed the worker can move forward in the confidence that change in
one area will have a 'ripple effect' in others. However, if, as Vickery's
text suggests, some systems in the case are more responsible than others
for holding Family X in its present state, their relative strengths must
be assessed. Change by psychiatric treatment does not seem to have
worked. Accepting the view that the unfriendly neighbourhood and lack
of support from friends and relatives are the more powerful factors, the
worker still has quite an array of alternative systems in the whole configuration with which intervention might be effective.

Internal Characteristics: Psychological and Sociological. Although a
systems approach tends to focus attention on the transactions among
systems, this is not to underestimate the importance of a system's internal state and relationships. Viewed as systems, individual human beings
have a variety of internal properties, and so do groups and organisations. These include needs, aims, sources of strain, habitual responses to
strain and ways of coping with responses to strain.[39] In personality
systems these variables have a psychological meaning, and in social
systems a sociological meaning. As Chaiklin[40] points out, this distinction
is important since it helps the social worker to avoid reductionist thinking and to choose appropriately between a psychological and a socio-

logical frame of reference. Vickery illustrates this point by the case of the conflict of values between father and son.[41] The worker who works with either the father or the son on his own must discuss the problem from a psychological intrapersonal viewpoint. If the worker works with son and father together or with the family as a whole, he is working in the interpersonal realm of value conflict and requires a social/psychological analysis.

System Regulating Processes. Both personality and social systems have varying degrees of need to maintain themselves. Sometimes the concepts of 'homeostasis' and 'equilibrium' are used to denote the tendency of a system experiencing tension and conflict to react in such a way as to bring it back to a former conflict-free and tension-free state. For some kinds of systems in certain contexts this is undoubtedly the case, but for others the maintenance of the system requires enduring change in response to changing environmental circumstances. How can the system change and at the same time remain essentially the same? The concept of the 'steady state' is sometimes used to denote the way in which systems achieve this. Goldstein states it thus:

'It is not the structure of the system that remains steady, for in order to maintain wholeness and continuity, some alteration of that structure may be a consequence of the system's endeavour to deal effectively with the inflow of stimuli. The superordination of roles, the reordering of performances, and the inclusion or exclusion of its members are structural changes that may be attendant to the system's attempts to sustain healthy stability, to mature and unfold.'[42]

This last point is important since there is a tendency to equate the use of systems theory with a view of man in society that is intolerant of conflict and that resists the breaking up of some systems for the sake of others. Some desirable changes, however, require that the system survive. Goldstein writes:

'The concept of a social system encourages a fluid and responsive approach – one which sensitises the social worker to the immediate ramifications of changes in the composition and balance of the particular system. His aim is to foster change and at the same time attend to the conditions which permit that system to retain enough equilibrium to manage that change.'[43]

Social Systems and a Unifying Framework. We have touched rather superficially on a few properties of a systems approach that offer new perspectives of old and familiar ground. These can be used in many different ways ranging from micro- to macro-systems, and within different theoretical frameworks. However, in providing a unifying framework their chief merit lies in their capacity to bring into focus a wide variety of social systems and variables of which the practitioner takes account. While this wider range may seem to add to the complexity of problem situations, it also may offer greater promise of effecting change.

As a unifier of social work practice the use of a social systems approach is compelling. Even authors like Maas[44] and Spergel,[45] who make the problem situation the unifying focus, inevitably emphasise the inter-relations between the client system and other systems impinging on it and they argue that the identification of worker activity with a particular size of client system is neither helpful nor real. Optimally, all workers relate to and try to influence individuals, organisations, families and groups irrespective of the type and size of their client system. Knowledge of and skill in relating to organisations and groups is as important for the caseworker as knowledge and skill in relating to individuals and families is for the community worker. This truth is the foundation of the unitary method.

Two Models of a Unitary Approach

We have already referred to the two texts that offer a unitary approach to social work practice, one by Pincus and Minahan, and the other by Goldstein. Pincus and Minahan have contributed a summary of their work to this volume (Chapter 5), and Goldstein has contributed a paper in which he describes how he came to develop his unitary approach and the way in which social systems theory is useful to social work practice (Chapter 4). We will now identify a few of the salient features of their textbooks on unitary method.

In neither text do the authors claim to have incorporated all the knowledge of practice that a caseworker, group worker and community worker might bring together. On the contrary they each delineate the boundaries of their content.

Goldstein, in his introduction, sets out four levels of knowledge ordered in increasing order of specificity and utility for social work practice: (1) the level of general concepts, such as theories of personality and the social order, which serve to provide broad understandings of certain phenomena in conceptual and hypothetical terms; (2) functional concepts such as group dynamics and aspects of communication theory that make phenomena accessible to manipulation; (3) the level of 'strategies', such as study and evaluation, which offer guides to the application of knowledge to given situations; and (4) the level of 'actions' which are the specific tactical procedures employed in specific situations. He states that his text stays on the second and third levels of functional concepts and strategies. He assumes the reader will have access to learning in the first level and the opportunity to participate in the realities of practice in the fourth level (Introduction, p. xii).

Pincus and Minahan state that their text is to serve as an introductory course. It is not their intention to provide a base for a generalist practitioner as opposed to a specialist. Rather it is a foundation on which the practitioner can build further knowledge as he chooses (Preface, p. xiii).

The authors' structural frameworks for social work practice are different but each text is embedded in systems theory. As we have already noted, Pincus and Minahan use it implicitly, and Goldstein uses it explicitly. He has a whole chapter on the client viewed as a system within a network of inter-related systems, any of which might be appropriate for intervention. He also gives considerable attention in another chapter to the individual social worker as a system within a change system that includes the agency system, the worker and the client system. This gives great richness to the reader's understanding of all the factors that make up the worker–client relationship and that determine its nature and outcome.

Pincus and Minahan give less detailed attention to the description of the structure of the social phenomena with which social work is concerned. But they define the functions of social work as they see them more specifically than Goldstein, thus giving more of a structure than Goldstein to the purposes of social work. They state that the purpose of social work is to enhance the problem-solving and coping capacities of people, to link people with systems that provide them with resources, services and opportunities, to promote the effective and humane operation of these systems and to contribute to the development and improvement of social policy. The main structural dimension of their practice model is their identification of four basic major systems: the client system, change-agent system, target system and action system; and they emphasise, as all system writers do, that it is not inevitable that the target system (i.e. the system that the worker and client decide to influence) and the client system be one and the same. For example, the client system in a particular case might be a single-parent family, the target system the department of health and social security, and the action system a 'gingerbread group' that includes the family's mother. This differentiation helps the worker to clarify the nature of his various relationships with and obligations to each of these systems.

Goldstein's model combines three major frameworks: the social systems model to which we have already referred; a social learning or problem-solving model; and a process model. The social learning or problem-solving model occupies a more all-embracing meaning than does Pincus and Minahan's discussion of the social work problem-solving process. They use as an example the familiar type of formula:

recognition and engagement with the problem, data collection, diagnosis, intervention, evaluation and termination. Like many other writers, they state that this is, in reality, not sequential in time, but rather a cyclical process recurring within a very short time span in each social work endeavour.

Goldstein, in explicating his model of social learning, devotes much more attention to this process and then places it within his third major framework, a process model of practice. Here he calls it a strategy of study and evaluation, intention and intervention, and appraisal; and he attempts to depict and describe it running through and recurring in different phases of the work process, namely, the role induction phase, the core phase and the ending phase of the work. He further breaks the whole process model down into types of targets: namely, individuals, families, groups, organisations and communities. Here, the concepts he has to use become more specific to the particular types of target system, and the reader becomes aware of the point at which greater theoretical specificity has to be introduced into a unitary model to take account of the different levels of analysis and theoretical frames of references that are required.

The major part of Pincus and Minahan's text is concerned with acquainting the reader with eight essential practice skills areas: assessing problems, collecting data, making initial contacts, negotiating contracts, forming action systems, maintaining and co-ordinating action systems, exercising influence and terminating the change effort. Having stated the cyclical nature of the analytical aspect of the problem-solving process, Pincus and Minahan clearly feel free to examine in detail each stage in a logical sequence of events without explicitly attempting to insert the problem-solving process within each one. The result is that for each stage they are able to draw on examples of practice in a wide variety of situations and they are less constrained than Goldstein by the need to be specific about the theoretical analysis of the structural system of each example.

In their section on practice skills, Pincus and Minahan give considerable attention to the forming, maintaining and co-ordinating of action systems. While not ignoring what this means in relation to work with individuals, it places an emphasis on the knowledge and skills required in work with groups. Here we catch a glimpse of the importance of this subject in relation to the development of a worker who, within a social systems configuration, can follow in practice as well as in theory where the logic of the problem analysis would take him.

In comparing the two texts there are many similarities in content even though it may be differently organised within the respective models. However, the general thrust is different. Pincus and Minahan are much concerned with the social worker's function of bringing client systems and resource systems into creative relationships with one another. While not diminishing the importance of appropriate resource acquisition and utilisation as a goal of social work, Goldstein is more concerned with the social worker's function of enhancing and intensifying focused social learning. He gives 'social learning' a very broad general meaning. He does not confine himself to individual or small group systems as being the main targets of change. He also sees larger systems as changing only through a social learning process. He writes:

'The assertion that change is ultimately lodged in persons is not incongruent with more sweeping or expansive emandations of larger systems. . . . We tend to abstract these phenomena, to see them in non-human, institutional, or societal terms as if they were occurring in a self-enclosed sphere. They are, in reality, human endeavours brought about by persons who are committed to the need for change, reform or modification. . . .' (p. 159).

Goldstein is quite explicit in his belief that social work should value equally the importance of what people learn as well as what they achieve. Extending, as he does, the social learning concept to cover learning in therapeutic endeavours as well as learning in social action endeavours, he avoids the value conflicts inherent, for example, in viewing client systems as requiring treatment and social institutions as requiring annihilation. He considers an educational, problem-solving approach to be one of the concepts that illustrate the emerging concurrence and unity that give the profession its own identity. This concept, he says, '. . . alludes to a common base of practice which, irrespective of the intent or purpose, conceives of social work as a means of providing new ways of perceiving and learning, new knowledge, access to a broader and more useful range of alternatives for action, and the opportunity to find out more productive types of social living' (p. 54).

Both Goldstein and Pincus/Minahan emphasise the importance of social problem-definition, and the assessment of where, within accessible social systems, intervention is required. This is the hall-mark of a unitary approach, and is in marked contrast to practice that is guided by the size of the client system with which the worker is concerned and with the problem or pathology it presents. But because Pincus and Minahan state more explicitly and give more space to goals such as linkages with resource systems, intervention within resource systems and the influencing of social policy, there seems to be a difference in the relative values placed on what is learnt and what is achieved in the social work process. The difference may be more apparent than real in that, as we have already indicated, Goldstein is dealing with social work practice at a higher level of abstraction than Pincus and Minahan. But even the possibility of conflict of values at a more operational level does not make invalid the notion of a unified profession or a common methodology. Controversy about goals and procedures is endemic in all professions. However, even with a common methodology, the question remains of how to organise knowledge about people, problems, situations, systems and their inter-relations for responsible action toward a specified end.

NOTES AND REFERENCES FOR CHAPTER 3

1 Isaiah Berlin, *The Hedgehog and the Fox* (London: Weidenfeld & Nicolson, 1967), pp. 7-8.
2 Max Siporin, 'Situational assessment and intervention', *Social Casework* (February, 1972), p. 109.
3 *Report of the Working Party on Social Workers in Local Authority Health and Welfare Services.*
4 See: ibid.; Chapter 6 in this volume; Anne Vickery, 'Specialist: generic: what next?', *Social Work Today*, vol. IV, no. 9 (26 July 1973); Noel Timms, *Language of Social Casework* (London: Routledge & Kegan Paul, 1968), ch. 5.
5 In 1919 the Institute of Almoners (Medical Social Workers) set up a course that added to existing social science content material necessary to almoners, and provided practical training.
6 Pauline C. Shapiro, 'Some "after care" patients in rural areas', *British Journal of Psychiatric Social Work*, vol. I, no. 2 (1947); E. M. Goldberg, 'The psychiatric social worker in the community', *British Journal of Psychiatric Social Work*, vol. IV, no. 2 (1957).
7 Eileen Younghusband, *Report on the Employment and Training of Social Workers* (Dunfermline: Carnegie United Kingdom Trust, 1947), para. 207(i).
8 *Report of the Committee on Local Authority and Allied Personal Social Services*, paras. 516-20.
9 ibid., para. 434.
10 ibid., para. 558.
11 *Report of the Working Party on Social Workers*, para. 949(e).
12 Eileen Younghusband, 'Social work in the future: trends and training', a talk at the New University of Ulster (June 1973; Chapter 6 in this volume).
13 Mary E. Richmond, *What Is Social Casework? An Introductory Description* (New York: Russell Sage Foundation, 1922), p. 102.
14 Robert D. Vinter, 'Essential components of group work practice', in *Readings in Group Work Practice* (Ann Arbor: University of Michigan, 1967).
15 Carole E. Holder, 'Temper tantrum extinction: a limited attempt at behaviour modification', *Social Work (UK)*, vol. XXVI, no. 4 (October 1969), pp. 8-11.
16 Tom Stephens (ed.), *Problem families: An Experiment in Social Rehabilitation* (Pacifist Service Units, 1945), pp. 45-66; A. F. Philp and Noel Timms, *The Problem of the 'Problem Family'* (Family Service Units, 1957), p. 38.
17 Neil Gilbert and Harry Specht, 'The incomplete profession', *Social Work* (New York; November 1974). See Chapter 13 in this volume.
18 Werner W. Boehm, 'Towards new models of social work practice', *Social Work Practice* (National Conference on Social Welfare; New York: Columbia University Press, 1967), p. 3.
19 David Donnison, *Social Policy and Administration* (London: Allen & Unwin,

1965), pp. 231–6; David Jones, 'Community work in the United Kingdom' (Chapter 10 in this volume).

20 Calouste Gulbenkian Foundation, *Community Work and Social Change* (London: Longmans, 1968).

21 Beulah Rothman and Catherine Papell, 'Social group work models', *Journal of Education for Social Work* (Autumn 1966; Chapter 8 in this volume).

22 David Jones, Chapter 10 in this volume.

23 Gilbert and Specht, 'The incomplete profession'.

24 Ann Hartman, 'The generic stance and the family agency', *Social Casework* (April 1974), p. 207.

25 Ruth R. Middleman and Gale Goldberg, *Social Service Delivery: A Structure Approach to Social Work Practice* (New York: Columbia University Press, 1974).

26 James Whittaker, *Social Treatment: An Approach to Interpersonal Helping* (Chicago: Aldine, 1974).

27 Henry Maas, 'Purpose, participation and education', in Lilian Ripple (ed.), *Innovations in Teaching Social Work Practice* (New York: CSWE, 1970), pp. 9–21.

28 ibid.

29 Gilbert and Specht, 'The incomplete profession'.

30 Maas, 'Purpose, participation and education,' p. 21.

31 Francis Purcell and Harry Specht, 'The House on Sixth Street', *Social Work*, vol. X, no. 4 (October 1965).

32 Vickery, 'Specialist: generic: what next?'

33 Patrick Goldring, *Friend of Family* (Newton Abbot: David & Charles; New York: Barnes and Noble Books, 1973).

34 Camberwell Council on Alcoholism, Annual Reports.

35 Gordon Hearn (ed.), *The General Systems Approach: Contributions Toward an Holistic Conception of Social Work* (New York: CSWE, 1968); Janchill, 'Systems concepts in casework theory and practice'; Ben A. Orcutt, 'Casework intervention and the problems of the poor', *Social Casework* (February 1973); Vickery, 'A systems approach to social work intervention'; Gerald Rubin, 'General systems theory: an organismic conception for teaching modalities of Social Work Intervention', *Smith College Studies in Social Work* (June 1973); Hartman, 'The generic stance and the family agency; Carol Meyer, 'Direct services in new and old contexts', in Kahn (ed.), *Shaping the New Social Work*.

36 Pincus and Minahan, *Social Work Practice*.

37 Goldstein, *Social Work Practice*.

38 Vickery, 'A systems approach to social work intervention'.

39 Neil J. Smelser and William T. Smelser, *Personality and Social Systems* (New York: Wiley, 1963), pp. 3–13.

40 Harris Chaiklin, 'Social system, personality system and practice theory', *Social Work Practice* (National Conference on Social Welfare; New York: Columbia University Press, 1969).

41 Vickery, 'A systems approach to social work intervention'.

42 Goldstein, *Social Work Practice*, p. 116.

43 Howard Goldstein, 'Theory development and the unitary approach' (Chapter 4 in this volume).

44 Maas, 'Purpose, participation and education'.

45 Spergel, 'A multi-dimensional model for social work practice'.

Chapter 4

THEORY DEVELOPMENT AND THE UNITARY APPROACH TO SOCIAL WORK PRACTICE*

Howard Goldstein

When one encounters new theories about social behaviour and social change, the natural tendency is to assume that these ideas emerged neatly formed as a result of a logical and orderly process of deliberation. What is seen, however, is only the end product, the final form of the theory, and not the process that was involved in its elaboration. This process is frequently a prolonged, erratic and sometimes distressing sequence of searches and trials which, if seen in its entirety, would reveal that its origins included either the thoughtful observation of some social or interpersonal situation or the pursuit of a solution to a perplexing problem; that is, at some point someone began to examine or question something, either by a deliberate act or by a reflective response to a puzzling condition. It can be noted parenthetically that observation and inquiry are not only the tools of the theorist but also the attributes of the creative and imaginative social worker who accepts that there are not final or simplistic explanations of human problems and that there is no optimal set of techniques that can be used to help resolve them.

Observation means something more than merely seeing; it is the open-minded scrutiny of the patterns of a series of events that is, in effect, directed towards a grasp of their meanings and relationships. What comes out of this endeavour is the comprehension of conditions that were formerly not perceived and a recognition of how they are connected and interdependent. Similarly, with the increasing use of systematic inquiry, old problems can come to be seen in a new light as a result of finding more relevant and effective ways of asking questions about them. Simply stated, the act and the art of theorising is the attempt to make sense out of complex, elusive social situations. As it applies to social work, it is not for the sake of knowledge alone but, of greater importance, for how this knowledge can contribute to more effective

* First published in *The Social Worker/Le Travailleur Social*, vol. XLII, nos 3–4 (1974), pp. 181–8.

practice. This is an endeavour that is not without some risk, however. As one moves toward new perceptions and solutions it becomes necessary to abandon or reformulate ideas and methods that once provided some order to and security within the intangibles of the practice experience.

The evolution of the unitary approach to social work practice was no exception to the processes described. Uncertainty and discomfort were the stimulus and observation and inquiry were the eventual means by which a reformulation of practice was set in motion. Like most case-workers some years back, I was faced with a peculiar dilemma. On the one hand, the relationship I was able to form with my client and the skill that I was able to bring to bear created a powerful and significant experience for this individual as well as for myself. It fostered trust and offered the security within which my client could attempt new ways of confronting barriers to a more productive and gratifying style of living. On the other hand, the potentials for change, based on the personality theories that I used to understand my client and make sense out of his behaviour and needs, were often not realised. It seemed that there were always some amorphous, undefined obstacles 'out there', apart from our closed relationship, that tended to get in the way of sought-for outcomes. Other members of the client's family apparently didn't understand the good things that were happening or conditions in the client's environment or community detracted from the task in which we were engaged; or still other social forces would intrude into this seemingly well-ordered process of change.

In addition, I began to suspect that the cloistered quality of our relationship provided me with only a meagre perspective of my client. I could grasp only that facet of his style of being that emerged in response to how he perceived me within the time-limited periods of our association. And, in some measure I had to rely on how he understood and reported his and others' behaviour and attitudes in other relationships and environments, reports that could only be self-validating and constricted. Hence, it was this limited and questionable data that provided the substance for critical diagnostic and planning decisions.

Over time, the dissatisfaction and frustration resulting from these limitations effected a search for a more penetrating way of comprehending the being and world of my clients. The first change was a gradual shift away from dominant intrapsychic notions that offered a rich, sometimes even an exotic, appreciation of the inner life of persons but tended to exclude conditions outside them. For example, the concept of 'resistance' did not sufficiently account for the many forces within and external to the individual that impeded change and growth. In some instances, I found that the client lacked the knowledge that was needed to make effective decisions about his life and act on them. In others, I came to face the fact that pernicious social conditions created too great an obstacle to growth and change, despite my client's desire to overcome them. And, I could not overlook the fact that at times, what appeared to be resistance on my client's part was, in reality, his confused and blocked reaction to his own lack of clarity or the ambiguous way I responded to him. Thus, my more parochial points of view were, in time, supplanted by constructs of human behaviour that took into account, first, the more immediate and less evolutionary interpretations of a person's actions and attitudes and, secondly, a perception of persons not only as entities but as interacting members of a variety of social relationships as well.

The former borrows from the phenomenological philosophies and lends weight to the principle that all behaviour is purposive. In this sense, persons can be understood by their actions in and reactions to specific situations. The behaviour and attitudes presented in these events serves as the most reliable indicator of a person's strivings, needs and perceptions. All else – ideas about what has been or how things came to be – are merely speculations, constructs that are in the head of the observer. These notions may well add to the elaboration of meaning; however, there is also the risk that their conjectural nature may detract from the goal of reliable understanding. The conception of behaviour as purposeful and adaptive in the immediate social context invites a way of thinking and seeing that, on one level, gives credence to the behaviour itself and on another, strives to understand the intentions of the acting person that underlie his behaviour. Hence, the study of the conduct of the harsh and punitive mother need not be restricted to the consideration of possible causative conditions – for example, rejection or deprivation in her early life. Instead, a more profound and relevant understanding can be achieved by striving to grasp, first, the immediate implications of her behaviour – how it affects her self-image, the stability of the family, the development of the child or how it places her in jeopardy. At the same time, it is necessary to know how these actions are manifestations of prevailing intentions, the means by which she attempts to master or cope with conflict, fear, doubt and the like. She may, for example, suffer from illness or lack of energy, be unable to control feelings or even be reacting to the strains of living with an incorrigible child. The significance of this approach lies in the fact that it guides the worker into the materiality of the client's real world and, in so doing, leads to responsive and relevant behaviour. As meaning emerges, an appropriate range of interventions and priorities follows. The social worker might search for significant past information, impose needed controls, offer guidance or engage in other actions that are sensitively responsive to the client's actions and their purposes. In any case, a more responsible form of practice is assured – one that rests more on observations that can be validated than on rhetorical assumptions that cannot be rooted in the real world of the person.

As it became apparent that it was possible to deal with the empirical aspects of my client's social world, then I could begin to make use of the concepts coming out of the work of social and behavioural sciences that provided access to the interpersonal and transactional meanings of behaviour. Foremost amongst these were the number of still-viable role theories that characterise persons as versatile actors who enact a number of distinct roles on a variety of social stages. What differentiates role theory from other more unidimensional orientations is the factor of expectation – i.e. each social situation poses a somewhat different set of presumptions about how the person is to act within it. On the one hand, this approach opens to view the manner in which the individual perceives the specific situation and how he thinks he ought to behave within it. On the other, it reveals something about the characteristics of others in the person's proximal world as it points to their motives and expectations and how they influence and shape his role behaviour. Returning to our fictional punitive mother, we can now, through the use of role theory, also understand how she interprets her role as a mother and, as important, how others (her child, husband, other institutions) set up expectations for her. Further, we can see if there is any measure of concordance between these varied sets of expectations and their ramifications. Consideration of possible interventions to remedy the situation now becomes broadened to include their implications for all who have an investment in this mother's role. For example, the worker may envisage certain goals that are in themselves realistic for the mother *per se*, but may run counter to the expectations of others in her environment and therefore invite obstructive reactions.

As these new approaches fell into place and became part of my professional repertoire they, in turn, led to the likelihood of using other related concepts. One, linked directly to the phenomenological-adaptive idea, was the concept of motivation, the product of the investigations of psychologists and learning theorists. These findings propose that motivation is a dynamic rather than static force that explains how and why people erect barriers to learning and change. Instead of labelling persons who do not willingly enter into the change experience as 'hard-to-reach' or 'unmotivated', it encourages the study of the value or need factors that affect or block participation. It is assumed that persons are motivated to act or not to act by their needs or preferences at a particular point in time; thus the difficulty might not be an absence of motivation as such, but the fact that the social worker and the client may hold widely divergent perceptions of what needs to be changed and when. On still another dimension, theories of motivation illuminate the possible blocks to problem solving that bear on the capacities and skills that the client brings to the endeavour. If change is seen as a process that aims at the resolution of a set of problems that involves the combined and co-operative efforts of the client and the practitioner, then the client needs to be helped to overcome the obstacles that impede his effectiveness in how he begins to confront his problems. One client, therefore, may be mired in his particular state of apathy because he cannot envisage suitable goals; another may not be able to act because he lacks the support of others in his life; and still a third may be incapacitated because, although troubled by a problem, he cannot see the cause-and-effect relationships that continue to contribute to its existence. Hence, this theory precludes the short-circuiting of the change possibilities by attributing a negative label to the client. Instead, it encourages a search for the maladaptive factors that impede progress and, in themselves, require resolution even before work on the problem can begin.

Another premise directly complementing the conception of role as a social force was communication theory. In focusing on the transactions of persons in relation, it attempts to explain how persons present themselves in social situations and convey their self image, how they define their relationships with others, and how they designate their own and others' roles within these relationships through verbal and non-verbal interchange. This orientation enables the practitioner to become a participant-observer and to grasp not only the needs and motives of the communicator in interaction but also the techniques and styles that are used to express them. For example, the silent client is no longer seen in terms of the discomfort that he injects into the change experience; instead, his silence could come to be understood as an expression possibly of fear, avoidance, confusion or self-disqualification.

These new ways of seeing and understanding directly affected the nature of my practice and provided me with a greater range of alternatives for the way I could work with each client/problem situation. My work with individuals on a one-to-one relationship was determined by planful choice and not by the limitations of my method. The ability to perceive the individual as inseparable from his larger social relationships and contexts enabled me to work with families – particularly when it was apparent that the conflict we were attempting to resolve was, indeed, embedded in the complex network of family interaction. Practice with groups also followed as a means of directly confronting the intricacies of social behaviour that were not revealed or were not subject to challenge or resolution within the limited confines of the worker–client relationship. And, as I became more aware of the even more external strains and pressures that impinged on my clients and other members of the community, I was impelled to rethink what I, as a social worker, could accomplish within the walls of my office and agency. Entry into community action and development endeavours followed, a move abetted by what I learned from my clients as victims of larger social problems.

These changes, by and large, resulted from the pragmatic needs and experiences of day-to-day practice. Another dimension of my professional activity was my teaching role in the university. In attempting to transmit to graduate students reliable knowledge about the fundamentals of professional practice, I found, with other colleagues, that we were not achieving the desired coherence of instruction. This occurred in a programme that was initially constructed according to traditional conceptions of practice that assumed that effective practice could be partialised into the three methods that have characterised social work – casework, group work and community organisation and development. One of the many supports for this assumption was the literature that was available to the educational endeavour; most articles and books could be classified by their particular methods orientation.

Despite the many supports for a tri-method orientation, something in the educational event seemed to make the reality of the methods approach to practice and their separateness somewhat obscure. A suggestion of redundancy crept into the content of the three courses; as instructors, we found ourselves saying the same things in these courses although in different terms. Both formally and informally, we first began to question and examine what it was that caseworkers, group workers and community organisers were doing in their role responsibilities (again, the availability of role concepts made it possible to study the multiple personifications of the same entity). Obviously, the three functioned under the single mantle of the values, goals and identifications of the profession in its response to its social mission in society. Despite the use of the concepts of group, neighbourhood, community and organisation to define the target of practice, in the final analysis most professional services were aimed at or were designed to assist individuals either singularly or as interacting members of larger orders. A group or community is, after all, an abstraction of reality that succeeds in taking on substance only when each is defined by the characteristics of the persons that comprise each unit and the way they transact their business with one another. Hence, if we talk about the effectiveness or the movement of a group, we are, in essence, referring to the behaviour, needs, motivations and attitudes of identifiable persons in concert. When we allude to a community not just as a geographic configuration, we are indicating the existence of persons in proximity who have certain sets of needs, share or have conflict about certain social values, lead or follow, and live under a similar range of circumstances. Each person will individually experience the consequences of any change endeavour, whether it derives from social planning, legislation or modifications of institutions.

Then why the discrepancy in approaches to the resolution of social problems? Again it is a matter of cognitive vision – how what we know limits or directs what we can come to understand. Recently, walking the ocean's shore, I came upon a peculiar cluster of rocks. I was fascinated not only by their beauty and texture but also because they were so startlingly different from other rocks that I had seen before. If I had had the knowledge of a geologist I would have known immediately that they were of the igneous variety and could have told something about the erosive quality of the environment. Were I a local fisherman, I would have known whether I might find some mussels nearby. And if I had the eye of an artist I would have seen how the rocks reflected light and how I might reproduce their strange composition.

In much the same way, persons who identify themselves as caseworkers, group workers or community workers tend to apprehend the same human event in quite different frames of reference. As the caseworker relies on particular personality theories to organise his understanding, he is able only to perceive the internal or proximal conditions of the individual in his particular situation. Depending on the theories of group process that he uses, the group worker would strive to realise the meaning of multiple human interactions according to concepts of cohesion, norms, social climate, process and the like. The community organiser would frame his perceptions in accord with sociological or social psychological principles and explain an event in terms of constituencies, power, structure and function. This is not to derogate the value of these illustrative knowledge structures which are used to capture and make sense out of an event. It is doubtful at this point in the development of social knowledge that descriptions of human experiences and the social structure in which they occur can be fitted into a uniform set of abstractions. What is pointed to are the constraints of social theories. Despite their respective value, each theory only accounts for special aspects and fragments of a complex social event and is, of necessity, reductionistic.

These observations led to the inference that the definition of social work practice based on three separate methods was probably specious and, indeed, reflective of three different modes of perceiving and explaining. This assumption was further strengthened by the realities of practice – the demands that graduating social workers were encountering when they entered employment. Caseworkers found themselves working with groups and families as part of their responsibilities and, not infrequently, engaged with boards and citizen groups to resolve pressing issues bearing on the community or the operation of their agencies. Group workers learned that if their groups were effective, individual needs and concerns would surface and require their attention. Community organisers found the use of groups as a most effective medium for implementing their tasks. In addition, they needed interviewing skills to strengthen motivation, induce participation or deal with dissidents in order to generate planning and change. These are, of course, issues that still prevail.

These inferences resolved themselves over time into two inter-related assumptions that, in conceptual terms, verified what I found in direct practice: the first, that persons, individually or in concert, can best be known by their immediate behaviours and attitudes and, in turn, that these factors reveal values, needs and typical adaptations to their world; the second, that individuals can be known both as unique beings in their own right and simultaneously as integral elements of some larger social structure. Conversely, these larger systems – families, groups, neighbour-hoods and communities – needed to be seen both as complex entities and as composites of individual beings – each with his own needs, hopes and ambitions. The first directs one's sight to the significance of the present and the strains, strivings and meanings within it. The latter points to the relationships and transactions between smaller and larger social units. I found, however, that it was easier to apply these assump-tions to direct practice than it was to apply them to the educational enterprise. Although these ideas offered a more comprehensive outlook than did the single vision of the caseworker, the group worker or the community organiser, some unresolved division was still apparent; that is, it was now possible to sensitise the student who planned to work with individuals and families to the meaning and impact of larger systems. The student who intended to work with the latter could be made aware of the needs and motivations of individuals within these systems. Yet what was still lacking was a means of achieving a more holistic appraisal of the social problem needing attention, a way of over-coming an 'either/or' approach that would tend to circumscribe the limits of what the worker could do.

This state suggests the analogy of the photographer who, after endur-ing the frustration of attempting to record his world through the use of a single lens, now acquires two lenses – a telephoto and a wide angle. He sees his son playing in the midst of his summer garden and, proud of both, wants to capture the entire scene. Trying his telephoto lens, he finds that the stance, the freckles and the smile of his son are revealed vividly and in detail but only a suggestion of the beauty of the garden comes through. The other lens takes in the glow and colour of the scene but, in its breadth, loses much of the vitality contained within the glee in his son's smile. What is needed, then, is still another kind of optical system – one that captures the figure and the ground at once and, in so doing, accomplishes this end without loss to either. The counterpart of this need, for our purposes, would be a type of vision and understanding that takes in the whole of a social situation, delineates its significant parts and, most important, shows how these parts interact in a way that gives the whole its unique quality and character. This form of vision would achieve increased coherence among the strategies and techniques of the profession and place them in the service of the worker in response to his holistic appraisal of the problem or event.

Access to this form of perception and understanding was offered by social systems theory. Now, on the face of it, this appeared to be a rather formidable set of ideas. Borrowing general systems theory for application to human events (the social aspect) from its origins in the biological and physical sciences, one takes with it the accretion of terms that contribute to the construction of the systems model. These are, for example, systems boundaries, the concepts of equilibrium and steady state, input and feedback, convergence and differentiation (see Goldstein, *Social Work Practice*, for definitions). These are terms that are relatively foreign to the already burgeoning vocabulary of the profession and are, in addition, of a higher order of abstraction than the concepts that are usually employed in explaining human and social behaviour.

Some reflections about how social work has, in the past, borrowed knowledge from other disciplines gave some clues as to how social systems theory could be adapted to the needs of professionals. It seemed to me that the profession tended to embrace whole theories, schools and methods without sufficient discrimination. This resulted in a significant shift in the profession's course and commitments. In short, social work attempted to adapt to the theory rather than modifying the theory to fit the profession's goals (see Goldstein, *Social Work Practice*, for historical development). It is a given that social work is dependent on the social and behavioural sciences for substantive knowledge and in no way does this fact detract from the integrity of the profession. In providing the arena within which borrowed concepts and ideas could be applied to real life situations, it appeared that the particular task and contribution of the profession was the ability to integrate these pieces of knowledge, transform them into operational strategies and test their validity for the resolution of social problems. This function is evident in the recent maturation and sophistication of practice with groups – a result of the transformation of the products of the work of group dynamicists and social psychologists into definitive principles and strategies of practice.

The first step, then, in converting social systems theory into a set of principles for practice was to survey what relevance it had for the typical tasks of the social worker. It became apparent that the essence of the theory was the way that it simultaneously offered a view of order, relation and effect when applied to a social phenomenon. This provided the worker with a broader and more profound appreciation of the event and a wider range of options as to how he might intervene. The social worker concerned with the more extensive problems of housing, health or delinquency can, with the aid of social systems theory, take into account the characteristics and locations of pertinent institutions and organisations, affected populations, power sources, resources and so forth (order); he can then speculate about the linkages and/or blocks between these elements – e.g. the presence of interdependence or isolation, conflict or co-operation (relations); and, finally, he can make some valid assumptions about how change in any particular unit or sector of the system will have consequence for other parts (effect). Likewise, the worker confronted with a family problem would not be limited to a view of the family merely as a composite of individuals. In perceiving the family as a system he might, for example, characterise the family by the specific roles its members assume or have ascribed to them (order), by how these roles are acted out in interaction (relation) and by the possible implications for the balance of the family system if one or another of these roles changes in its potency (effect).

These examples point to the fact that systems theory is not a complex matrix that is universally or identically imposed on the varied conditions encountered in practice. It is a tool that can be modified to fit the problem. In each situation, the worker first constructs his notion of the system in his own mind. This depends on the range of circumstances and things that he needs to encompass relative to the task. He then enlarges or narrows his field and the targets within it as the relevant strategies and goals become apparent. Thus, the practitioner working with the more extensive problems of health or housing may find that he needs to expand his view of the apparent system to include, say, legislative bodies or governmental offices. Or, on the other hand, his analysis of the system may lead him to narrow his view and restrict his study to certain pertinent sub-systems – affected families, citizen groups and the like. These determinations do not occur by chance; instead, they are the product of the careful study of order, relation and effect in a given system. For example, awareness that the linkages between institutions and groups are tenuous might well urge the worker to direct his activities toward the engagement of the external, superordinate bodies to achieve change. Or the recognition that the potentiality for co-operation between certain groups is present may lead him to involve these groups in the change endeavour. The family social worker has the same options in determining whether he involves certain members of the family, the family as a whole or resources outside the family in the change process. This limited example of the use of systems theory may suggest that a fixed, unyielding process is set in motion much in the way that a programme is constructed for a computer. This is not the case; the concept of a social system encourages a fluid and responsive approach – one which sensitises the social worker to the immediate ramifications of changes in the composition and balance of the particular system. His aim is to foster change and at the same time attend to the conditions which permit that system to retain enough equilibrium to manage that change.

Beyond its instrumental value, the concept of social systems had the effect of redefining the social work role and task. It has been shown, first, that this more comprehensive approach to the study of social problems has led to a diffusion of the apparent boundaries between the traditional social work methods. Second, and of greater importance, it moves thinking forward toward a definition of practice in general that rests on the viable constructs of a problem-solving approach.

What is meant by a problem-solving approach? The very process of the study of a system is a prime example of a problem-solving enterprise. This study does not start out with fixed assumptions about the event but, instead, attempts to sort out factors that are related to it, determines their implications for one another, reconstructs the event into a more organic whole and, out of this endeavour, arrives at alternatives that can be tested. In its more usual forms, problem solving is an essential part of effective everyday living – in meal preparation, in planning for a vacation or in getting a stalled car started. In professional practice, problem solving takes on more planful and purposive characteristics as it requires more specialised knowledge and skills as well as a set of principles that will guide effective activity. This can be seen in the following series of steps that portray the problem-solving component of the practice experience.

(1) The social worker enters the problem situation equipped with a knowledge base and an array of strategies that he can call on as well as knowledge about other resources available to the task at hand. These capabilities can be used selectively and responsively as (2) an appraisal of the problem, its dimensions and implications, and the field within which it is located is made. Within this study (3) the social worker, with the mutual participation of the client system, sorts out what is most cogent, and surveys the relevant persons, groups or organisations that are affected by the conditions, contribute to them and have the potentiality for change. This process leads to (4) the determination of possible goals – both interim and long range. The resultant decisions about direction then recommend (5) possible strategies and alternatives for action. These are then rehearsed and tested within both the change experience and the locations of the problem. What emerges out of this occasion is (6) validation of the new endeavour, awareness of strengths and capabilities and transfer of what has been learned to other problem situations.

This model is, of course, an oversimplification of the complex process of human and social change within which allowances must be made for the fact that change does not take place at an even and orderly rate.

However, it does represent the essence of a planned change event. In so doing, it points to the transactional rather than the unilateral factors in problem resolution, a process that intends to involve the client system in all of its stages. Can we conclude, therefore, that the aim of helping is not only the solution of the apparent problem but, more important, facilitating the client systems' ability to develop the problem-solving capabilities required for the task as well as for other problems in living?

What we have arrived at as a consequence of inquiry and the analysis of practice is not a new social work practice but, instead, an explication and reformulation of what practice has been and can be. The concepts discussed in this paper do not negate existing orientations to practice; instead, they offer a comprehensive way, a framework, for organising what we do in practice and achieving a greater sense of purpose and accountability in our efforts.

Lastly, and perhaps most important, a systems orientation gently nudges the profession of social work into line with the inexorable recognition that all problems – political, economic, ecological as well as social – can no longer be understood in unidimensional terms. It becomes increasingly apparent that the neat compartments of the knowledge disciplines are eroding as the realisation grows that there are linkages between all events. The attempt to treat any one condition as if it were isolated from others results in fragmentation at best and in counter-productivity at worst. That this is an emerging realisation is evident in the number of new words that have found their way into the popular vocabulary – terms such as biophysics, geo-politics, psycho-biology and ecology – all pointing to the transactional character of phenomena. Social work literature now also reflects this shift. Ideas about 'mental illness' and 'psychopathology' which locate the source of dysfunction within the head of the patient are being reconsidered with the use of concepts of deviance. These take into account the impact of societal, cultural and institutional forces that influence ideas about who is considered aberrant as well as how, when and in what circumstances. We have come to understand population areas not merely as geographic or political entities but as organic communities that can be characterised by the complex of social values, groups and institutions that comprise them.

SUMMARY

This attempt to describe the development of the unitary approach to social work practice has two purposes. The first is to particularise and depict the steps that occurred and also to sort out and identify the concepts and theories that were employed, to show how they were built into the formulation, and to illustrate how they are useful for professional practice.

The second purpose is somewhat more implicit yet no less important. It is to demonstrate that theory development is, in itself, a learning and problem-solving process that is designed not only to resolve existing problems but also to open new approaches to the resolution of others. It is a process that begins with some concern, discomfort or puzzlement about an event or condition. This state, in turn, leads to a closer scrutiny and a restructuring of questions about the circumstances (e.g. why traditional casework techniques were not more effective). As the problem is defined, other more cogent kinds of information are sought and become apparent (e.g. social systems theory). New alternatives are suggested as the information is incorporated and they are activated. These new approaches to the problem are tested for their applicability to the resolution of human problems and are then refined into a set of principles used to guide subsequent behaviours. Over time, the results are then applied to other problem situations and the process continues. Theory building never reaches a final conclusion; instead, each formulation of ideas must be seen as one in a series of step functions – each leading to another. Thus, the intent of devising a unitary approach was not to offer a final statement about the nature of social work practice but to contribute to its continued growth and development.

Chapter 5

A MODEL FOR SOCIAL WORK PRACTICE

Allen Pincus and Anne Minahan

INTRODUCTION

This chapter will present a model – a way of describing social work practice. The model developed out of our experiences over a five-year period in developing and teaching social work practice at the School of Social Work at the University of Wisconsin-Madison in the United States. The model is described in detail in our book *Social Work Practice: Model and Method*.[1] Although our practice and teaching experiences have been primarily in North America, we believe social workers in many countries perform similar functions and tasks and thus hope our ideas may be useful to practitioners and teachers in Great Britain and other nations.

We began our search for a model of practice because of the limitations of describing social work according to its traditional three divisions of casework, group work and community organisation. We found it difficult to accept the thinking implied in each of the traditional methods – that social workers specialise in working with one size of system – individual, small group or community. We knew that caseworkers work with families and other groups, group workers with individuals, community workers with individuals and groups, and that all social workers work with organisations and segments of communities.

In developing our model we began by examining the tasks of the social worker in action as he works to change elements in a social situation in order to achieve a specified goal or outcome. Our model grew by bits and pieces as we isolated and identified basic elements in practice that were reflected in these tasks. We borrowed from existing formulations in the literature.

As our model grew, so did our conviction that regardless of the many forms social work practice takes, there is a *common core of concepts, skills, tasks and activities* which are essential to the practice of social work and represent a base from which all social workers can build. However, we want to emphasise that *our model does not provide a base for a generalist practitioner as opposed to a specialist.* It can set the foundation for either one, depending on how the practitioner builds on it. The social worker may incorporate into the model special knowledge about particular social problems (e.g. poverty, mental retardation), client groups (e.g. ageing, delinquents), organised societal systems (e.g. schools, hospitals), theoretical orientations (e.g. learning theory, social action) and organisation tasks and processes (e.g. administration, supervision).

Finally, we emphasise that our model is designed to provide a common base of knowledge, values and skills for professional social workers in any organisation that delivers services to people or in any field of practice. We assume people in any society need help with problems in social functioning. Although different societies have organised their response to these problems in diverse ways, we believe professional social workers are needed to perform essential functions in many societies. We will discuss the social conditions that are of concern to social workers and the purpose and function of social workers in the following section.

To place our model in context, we will first discuss our view of the nature of social work practice. The second section of the chapter will present several key concepts for analysing the activities of the social worker in action. The practice skills utilised by the social worker in carrying out his activities will be the focus of the third part of the chapter. Finally, we will end with some general observations about our model.

NATURE OF SOCIAL WORK PRACTICE

Resource Systems

The focus of social work practice is on the interactions between people and systems in their social environment. People are dependent on social systems for help in obtaining the material, emotional or spiritual resources and the services and opportunities they need to realise their aspirations and to help them cope with their life tasks. By life tasks we mean the responses people make as they face the demands made upon them in various life situations such as growing up in a family, entering school or work, marrying, raising a family, and facing illness and death.[2]

In some societies, the family or the tribe are the major systems that provide people with the resources they need to help them cope with their life tasks. However, in industrialised and bureaucratic societies, people have become dependent on help from extra-family resources such as places of work, schools and units of government; and these systems have become complex and often difficult to negotiate.

People in many countries today can find help from three kinds of resource systems: (1) *informal or natural resource systems* consisting of family, friends, neighbours, co-workers, bartenders and other helpers; (2) *formal resource systems* which may be membership organisations or formal associations such as labour unions or neighbourhood associations which promote the interests of their members; and (3) *societal resource systems* such as schools, hospitals, housing authorities, police departments and financial assistance agencies.

Despite the help potentially available from the network of informal, formal and societal systems, there are situations in which people are unable to obtain the resources, services or opportunities they need to cope with their life tasks and realise their aspirations. Existing systems may be inadequate for many reasons: (1) a needed resource system may not exist or may not provide appropriate help to people who need it; (2) people may not know a resource system exists or may be hesitant to turn to it for help; (3) the policies of the resource system may create new problems for people; or (4) several resource systems may be working at cross-purposes.

In addition to these inadequacies, any one of the systems may not be functioning properly because of internal problems that hamper its effectiveness. A family, a membership organisation or a societal system may be hampered by internal conflict between its members, inadequate procedures for making decisions and solving problems or faulty internal communications. Thus the internal functioning of the systems established to help people meet their life tasks and realise their values and aspirations may be the cause of problems for people within the system. It may also keep the systems from aiding people who come to them for help.

Functions of Social Work Practice
In dealing with such situations described above we observe social workers performing a variety of functions.

(1) Helping People Enhance and More Effectively Utilise Their Own Problem-solving and Coping Capacities. The social worker performs this function with people who cannot cope with their life tasks and may experience distress because of physical, emotional, economic or social problems. These problems may prevent an individual, who could be connected to several systems (family, place of work, school), from functioning satisfactorily within them. Individuals may also be so overwhelmed and confused by the life tasks facing them that they may need help in establishing realistic goals and aspirations for themselves and in deciding what they can do to achieve them.

(2) Establishing Initial Linkages between People and Resource Systems. Social workers need to perform this function because people who need resources may not be linked to informal, formal or societal systems

because they may not know of their existence or how to use them, because they may be reluctant to use the systems or believe they will not meet their needs, or because a needed resource system does not exist.

(3) Facilitating Interaction and Modifying and Building New Relationships between People and Societal Resource Systems. After initial linkages have been formed between people and societal resource systems, problems may occur which prevent societal systems from being responsive to their consumers and keep people from receiving the help they need. Indeed, the nature of the interactions between people and resource systems may aggravate rather than reduce problems, or may create new problems. The social worker needs to facilitate interactions between systems for several reasons: (*a*) the operation of some societal systems actually dehumanises the people they were established to serve; (*b*) some societal systems are unresponsive to those who come to them because members of the societal system and consumers disagree as to the nature of the problems and what should be done about them; (*c*) within large societal resource systems such as hospitals or schools, people may not be receiving all the appropriate services the systems can provide; (*d*) if consumers are receiving services from several sub-parts of a societal system, or from many societal systems, they may find that these systems are working at cross-purposes.

Of course, many of the social worker's activities in performing this function are designed to make his own societal system responsive to its consumer.

(4) Facilitating Interaction and Modifying and Building Relationships between People within Resource Systems. In contrast to the last function which focuses on worker's activities in changing interactions *between* people and resource systems, this function highlights the activities of the worker aimed at changing the interactions of people *within* an informal, formal or societal resource system in order to enable the system to meet the needs of its members and, in the case of societal resource systems, to improve their ability to provide resources for their consumers.

The worker may be seeking to help family members change the way they relate to each other, to help them provide emotional support and affection for one another, to help members of a neighbourhood association deal with problems of internal dissension or to help staff members of a hospital redefine their working relationships. In all these situations, the worker's activities are directed toward helping individual members of the system carry out their roles within the system, as well as improving the operation of the system as a whole.

In working to change transactions between people in a resource system, the worker operates on the assumption that if he helps the system to provide satisfaction for its members, the system will be better able to achieve its goals. Types of problems that may hamper the functioning of a system include apathy, conflict between members, poor communication, and inadequate procedures for making decisions and solving problems. Further, the distribution of power and authority in the system and conflicting values among members may prevent some members from achieving satisfaction in their roles.

The worker may be a member of the system he is trying to help or outside it. The worker within his own societal system may or may not have formal administrative responsibility, but he is responsible for trying to change faulty functioning of his system that prevents it from serving in the best interest of its consumers.

(5) Contributing to the Development and Modification of Social Policy. Social workers work for changes in social policies that affect people in many informal, formal and societal resource systems. Thus social workers contribute to the development and modification of social policy made by legislative bodies, elected heads of government, public administrative agencies, voluntary funding institutions and people in positions of authority in societal resource systems.

Social workers, often in co-operation with others, work for many social policy objectives. They call attention to unmet needs and gaps in present resources and dysfunctional aspects of existing social policy and legislation. Social workers help design and promote the establishment of new services, co-ordinate and integrate existing societal resource systems and work to influence and sometimes help shape social policy and legislation designed to alter the social conditions and restraints under which people live.

All of the functions discussed above are designed to alleviate problems in the interactions between people and systems in their social environment. In addition to these functions, in many societies social work has performed two other vital societal functions: dispensing material resources and serving as an agent of social control. Many societies have sanctioned the performance of these functions by social workers, in co-operation with other professions and occupations. Social workers have accepted these functions and developed competence in performing them. Social workers who perform these essential societal functions bring to their performance their particular perspective and skills in improving the interactions between people and their social system. However, we believe the performance of these functions is not, and should not be, the central core or focus of social work.

(6) Dispensing Material Resources. Social workers dispense material resources – money, food, adoptive and foster homes, and other resources

that are crucial for people's survival. Ordinarily when social workers dispense material resources, they are operating as agents not only of a social agency but also of society. They are bound by legislative and agency mandates, regulations and standards. In addition, social workers themselves have developed professional standards of practice in this area, such as in the fields of foster care and adoption.

(7) Serving as Agents of Social Control. Some societal systems have been granted the authority to serve as agents of social control for people whose behaviour deviates from societal laws and norms and to protect people who may be harmed by the behaviour of others. Societal systems exercise their authority to confine people whose behaviour has been labelled deviant, in prisons, mental hospitals and other institutions. They also supervise people in the community who have committed deviant acts, remove children and other dependent people (severely mentally retarded or physically handicapped) from situations where they may be harmed, and establish and enforce standards for care of dependent people. Social workers who serve as agents of social control receive their sanction and authority through their employment in societal resource systems.

Social workers perform a variety of activities and tasks to accomplish one or more of the seven functions of social work.[3] These tasks may involve the workers in activities designed to advocate, educate, facilitate or organise new systems. The worker uses social work knowledge and concepts to aid him in selecting appropriate tasks and activities and social work skills in performing these tasks.

Purpose of Social Work
As we examine the nature of the problem situations social workers address themselves to and the functions they perform in dealing with such situations, a definition of social work and a frame of reference for its operation begin to emerge.

Our definition of social work practice focuses on the *linkages* and *interactions* between people and resource systems and the problems to be faced in the functioning of both individuals and systems. The definition is:

Social work is concerned with the interaction between people and their social environment which affects the ability of people to accomplish their life tasks, alleviate distress and realise their aspirations and values. The purpose of social work therefore is to (1) enhance the problem-solving and coping capacities of people, (2) link people with systems that provide them with resources, services and opportunities, (3) promote the effective and human operation of these systems and (4) contribute to the development and improvement of social policy.

Social Work Frame of Reference

Social work has developed a frame of reference which reflects its purpose and provides it with a unique way of viewing and dealing with social situations.

First, in viewing a social situation, the social worker's concern is with the life tasks confronting people and the resources and conditions which would facilitate their coping with these tasks, help them realise their values and aspirations and alleviate their distress. For example, consider a family in which one of the children is mentally retarded. The concern of social work here is not with the mental retardation *per se* but with the tasks that having a mentally retarded child present to the family and their ability to cope with these tasks. Do the parents have the knowledge and time to deal with any special problems the child might present? Are there resources in the community such as special day-care centres and schools? Are the parents aware of and able to use such resources? Is there an organised group of parents of mentally retarded children which could provide the parents with information and advice, help link them to needed resources as the child grows up, provide an outlet for sharing problems and concerns, and act as an advocate for their interests?

A second characteristic of the social work perspective on social situations is its focus on people in interaction with their network of resource systems. This means that we do not view problems as an attribute of people; rather, we see people's problems as an attribute of their social situation. The question is not who *has* the problem, but how the elements in the situation (including the characteristics of the people involved) are interacting to frustrate people in coping with their tasks. In this context social workers can define a problem as a social situation or social condition which has been evaluated by someone as undesirable. In this view, no social situation is in itself inherently a problem. When a situation is referred to as a problem, it must be realised that an implied evaluation of it has already been made. If we accept this definition, a problem can be seen as constituting a cluster of three related parts: (1) a social condition or social situation, (2) people who are evaluating the social condition or situation as problematic and (3) the reasons or bases for their evaluation.

Most situations confronting a social worker involve looking at three types of interaction: among people within a resource system (informal, formal or societal), between people and resource systems, and between resource systems. Consider a social worker in a community centre who is asked to help a low-income family with young children who are having difficulty in school. The social worker's assessment of the situation would include the problems within the family, the problems the children are having in the school and the problems the school is having in teaching these and other low-income children. The goals of the social worker, to help the family and the school improve the ways they deal with each other, may call for intervention on several levels: (1) influencing the school to change its transactions with this low-income family and other low-income children and families; (2) helping the individual family members improve the social interactions within the family to enable each family member to achieve his maximum growth; (3) helping the family to change its interactions with the school; and (4) helping the family and other community institutions to improve the ways they deal with each other.

The third aspect of the social work frame of reference directs the worker's attention to the relationships between the private troubles of people in a social situation and the public issues which bear on them. Many personal troubles cannot be dealt with by an individual or family because they are linked to public issues. Reciprocally, problems of public issues cannot be handled without examination of their impact on personal troubles.

To illustrate the relationship between personal troubles and public issues, consider the problems of health needs of elderly people. An aged person who needs but cannot find adequate nursing home care has a private trouble. However, the shortage of good quality nursing care and the existence of substandard nursing homes is a public issue. If social workers concentrate on helping individual aged people find scarce nursing home care, they are only dealing with private troubles. They cannot alleviate many of these private troubles, however, without also working on the public issue – the expansion of quality nursing home care. And, in order to substantiate the need for nursing home expansion and improvement, social workers must cite the need for such care by many individuals and describe the private troubles related to the public issue.

To summarise, the social work frame of reference leads the practitioner to focus on three related aspects of social situations: (1) the life tasks people are confronted with and the resources and conditions which would facilitate their coping with these tasks; (2) the interactions between people and their resource systems, as well as the interactions within and among resource systems; and (3) the relationship between the private troubles of people and public issues which bear on them.

PRACTICE CONCEPTS

Having presented a frame of reference for understanding the social phenomena with which social work is concerned we will now consider how to analyse the activities of the social worker in action. This section will present some key concepts for organising our thinking about how the social worker carries out his role. In the following section we will discuss the practice skills employed by the worker.

The Four Basic Systems

The key element of our model is a classification of the types of systems in relation to which the social worker carries out his role. One thing which becomes apparent when observing the activities of social workers is the variety of people and systems which they interact with in carrying out their work. This can be expected because of social work's concern with the interaction of people and resource systems. For example, a social worker in corrections works with probationers, their families, schools, employers, lawyers, courts, welfare departments and other community agencies. A social worker in a hospital works with patients, their families, doctors, nurses, other hospital staff, health clinics, visiting nurses and a host of other groups and agencies.

In understanding this array of relationships we are led to ask certain questions. Who is supposed to benefit from the worker's change efforts? Who has given him sanction for his work? Who is he trying to change or influence? Who is he working with to achieve different goals in his change efforts? We can begin to sort out such issues by identifying four types of systems in relation to which the worker carries out his activities.

Change Agent System. A social worker can be viewed as a change agent, and the public, voluntary or profit-making agency or organisation that employs him as a change agent system. We identify this system to emphasise that the worker is influenced in his change efforts by the system of which he is a part and which pays his salary. The social worker will be operating with different sanctions, constraints and opportunities when his own agency, as contrasted to an outside system, becomes a target for change.

Client System. The client system is the person, family, group, organisation or community which engages the services of the worker, establishes a working agreement (which we will refer to as a contract) with the worker and is the expected beneficiary of the worker's efforts. The working agreement or contract may be with the entire client system or some subpart of it (e.g. one member of a family, the board of directors of an agency, one organisation in the community). The social worker may attempt to enlarge the client system by involving other members of a larger system in the contract, or to reduce the client system by limiting his contractual agreements.

As the term is used here the client system is not necessarily the target of the social worker's interventions, although this is the sense in which the term is often used in social work. Sometimes in order to serve the client system we need to influence another system to change.

Social workers often work with people referred to as 'involuntary clients', i.e. persons who have not requested or contracted for our services. Initially a worker in protective services for children or corrections does not have a contract with the parent or prisoner. His initial sanction to engage in specific activities in these cases comes from the agency which employs him (the change agent system) and thus indirectly from the community which supports the agency. In such cases an important task of the worker is to influence such potential clients to become actual clients, thus shifting the source of his sanction from the community directly to those whom he seeks to work with.

The Target System. The 'target system' refers to those people the change agent needs to influence in order to accomplish the goals of his change effort.

An important diagnostic task of the social worker, usually in collaboration with the client system, is to establish the goals for change and then determine the specific people – the targets – that will have to be changed if the goals are to be reached. To illustrate, the neighbourhood worker may be asked by members of a group to help them achieve the goal of improving their housing conditions. The social worker agrees, and together they identify several targets: landlords, city housing inspectors, members of the city sanitation department and others. Some of these targets may agree readily to make changes; others may be recalcitrant and resistant or fight the change efforts. A point we want to emphasise again is that the client system is not always the system that needs to be changed (in other words, it is not always the target) in order to reach the change goals.

Sometimes the client system and the target system will be the same, as when a change agent accepts an individual client for help in solving a personal problem. In other cases, the client system may be considered the target system in working toward some goals, but in respect to other goals, the target and client systems may differ and be apart. In the example of the neighbourhood group trying to improve their housing, the group and the worker have identified target systems (inspector of the city sanitation department and landlords) outside the client system and asked the alderman and newspaperman to try to influence the targets. Members of the group also may want to talk directly with city officials but be afraid to present their problems in this way and lack confidence in their ability to gain access to these people and to present an effective case. The worker may need to give them encouragement and help them plan and rehearse what they will say. In this activity the worker views the members of the group as another target system, and his goal is not only to help them with their housing problems but also to enhance their feelings of self-worth and give them confidence which will help them deal with other problems and situations.

When the social worker seeks to change the policy makers in his own agency in order to provide better service for the community and his clients, the change agent system itself may become a target system.

In any one change effort, the social worker will identify several goals over a period of time. Thus different people may be considered targets for different goals at different times.

Action System. As indicated by the examples illustrating interactions between the change agent, client and target systems, the change agent does not work in isolation in his change efforts; he works with other people. The term 'action system' refers to the social worker and the people he works with and through to accomplish the tasks and achieve the goals of the change effort. An action system can be used to obtain sanctions and a working agreement or contract, identify and study a problem, establish goals for change or influence the major targets of change. In any one problem situation the change agent may work with several different action systems to accomplish different tasks and achieve different goals.

Depending on the situation, an action system could be:

(1) A new system put together by the worker with the expectation that the members of the system will be in direct interaction with each other. For example, a nursing home social worker could form a group of residents to plan activities and programmes or to give advice to the staff on operating the home.

(2) An existing system already in operation. Examples are a family with an alcoholic husband, or a teenage gang operating in the area of a neighbourhood centre.

(3) Several people who may not at any one time be engaged in direct interaction with one another but whom the worker will co-ordinate and work with to change a target on behalf of a client. For example, the probation officer may co-ordinate the activities of an employment office worker, employers, a welfare worker, a teacher at a vocational school and others in his work on behalf of the probationer.

Thus change agents may work with a number of different types of action systems at different steps in their change efforts.

Relationship

The relationships the worker forms with the people in the four systems described above are the medium through which he carries out his activities. Although social workers form different relationships with different systems, there are common elements in all professional relationships which differentiate them from personal relationships. These elements are: (1) purposefulness: relationships are formed for purposes related to the worker's planned change effort, (2) client focused: devoted to the client's interests, needs and aspirations rather than those of the worker and (3) objectivity: self-awareness which allows the worker to step outside his own personal troubles and emotional needs and to be sensitive to the needs of others. These aspects of a professional relationship have received much attention in the social work literature and are familiar to social workers. However, although social workers form relationships to achieve purposes related to the goals of the client system, there are important differences in social work relationships to achieve different purposes with different systems. A relationship can be thought of as an affective bond between the worker and other systems operating within a major posture or atmosphere of collaboration, bargaining or conflict. There has been a tendency in social work to view professional relationships as being synonymous with collaborative relationship. This is largely because of our preoccupation with focusing on relationships with client systems. But as our discussion of the four types of systems indicated, the social worker must be concerned with his relationships with all systems. While in practice every relationship contains elements of collaboration, bargaining or conflict, at any point in time a worker may be relating to another system essentially in one of these stances. Social workers must understand the factors that influence the kinds of relationships they work with and know how to operate within them.

Collaboration. Social workers normally have collaborative relationships with clients; indeed, the essence of forming a working agreement or contract with a client is for the social worker and the client to agree on the goals for the change process and the methods to achieve these goals. Collaborative relationships with clients are facilitated by social work values that stress self-determination and democratic decision making. People will more readily follow through on a change effort and, if necessary, take risks and make changes themselves, if they have sanctioned the change efforts, have helped establish the goals for change and have developed trust and confidence in the worker.

Collaborative relationships with clients who have problems of interpersonal social functioning have been described by many writers in terms of the change agent's creation of an accepting atmosphere by the way he relates to clients. This atmosphere promotes feelings of trust, genuineness and honesty between clients and workers.[4] Some writers on organisation and community change also stress the utility of collaborative relationships in working for change.[5] However, true collaborative relationships are possible only when there is agreement on the goals of the planned change effort and the methods for achieving the goals between the worker and his target system – those people the worker needs to change or influence in order to accomplish his goals.[6]

Interestingly, even if the worker believes his goals and the goals of his target are the same, if the target system *perceives* the goals as being different, or not in its self-interest, it may resist collaborative relationships.

Bargaining. When social workers make their first contact with a potential client, action or target system, the systems, in a sense, are in a bargaining relationship – each is testing the other to determine what the other's goals are, what demands will be placed on all parties and what the outcomes of the change efforts might be. If, after this initial testing, the conditions described above as amenable to collaborative relationships emerge, then a contract can be reached and collaborative relationships can follow.

A social worker becomes involved in bargaining relationships when: (1) there is a perceived difference between, on the one hand, the shared goals of the change agent and client systems and, on the other, those of the target system, (2) the target system perceives the change goals as not entirely in its self-interest, (3) the target system believes moderate demands for change will be placed on it and (4) conditions are present which force the parties into a bargaining situation where there is at least a possibility for agreement or accommodation.

In some bargaining situations, the social worker is bringing parties together to enable them to bargain, and in others the social worker himself is in a bargaining stance *vis-à-vis* another system. In the first case, the social worker may have collaborative relationships between himself and the individual bargainers and may be viewed by all concerned as a neutral, trustworthy mediator. In the second, the social worker is not neutral and may be seen as an advocate of a point of view trying to help a client system obtain something in the bargaining process. In the latter case, the social worker can be expected to use tactics of persuasion, negotiation and even confrontation – and, occasionally, guile – to enhance his bargaining position.

Conflict. If the bargaining relationships break down and the parties cannot reach agreement or accommodation, or if polarisation occurs between the perceived differences in the goals and demands of all parties, conflictual relationships may follow. They may also be inevitable if the shared goals of the change agent and client systems appear to pose a threat to the self-interests of the target system and are perceived by the target as requiring major changes in its functioning. Conflict is also likely to follow if the conditions that led to the establishment of a bargaining relationship were not present at the outset of the change effort, and if there appears to be no desire to negotiate differences.

The social worker thus faces situations when the use of conflictual relationships is required in order to achieve the shared goals of the worker and client system. A social worker acting on behalf of the community as client may have essentially a conflictual relationship with parents accused of child abuse. One working with an action and client system of neighbourhood residents may enter into conflictual relationships with landlords and city officials.

A social worker involved in conflictual relationships on behalf of his client system may not always operate with the expected social work values of openness, mutual trust and honesty *vis-à-vis* the target system. He may use such tactics as protest demonstrations, open confrontation, threats and court orders in his efforts to influence the target system, be it individual, group, or community organisation or institution.[7] However, few social workers advocate using tactics involving violence in a conflictual situation. Indeed, social workers are limited in their choice of intervention strategies by constraints that stem from the professional base of social work, from social work values, from the organisation that employs the social worker and from society.

Process
In addition to viewing the structure and nature of the change agent's working relationships, an understanding of the role of the social worker in action requires some concept to gain perspective on his activities over time, i.e. to view social work as a process.

It is useful to view social work as a planned change process. The word 'plan' conveys the idea of a purposeful and well-thought-out scheme, method or design for the attainment of some objective or goal. The word 'change' implies movement, a difference in or alteration of a situation or condition from one point in time to another. We view social work as a conscious, deliberate and purposeful planned change effort.

There are a number of descriptive and prescriptive models which divide the activities of a social worker in any planned change effort into predetermined sequential steps or phases. Each phase is characterised by some broad goal which must be accomplished before moving on to the next one.

For example, a study of the work of a variety of change agents such as social workers, psychiatrists and organisation consultants concludes that most change processes pass through the following seven phases:

(1) Development of a need for change.
(2) Establishment of a change relationship.
(3) Clarification or diagnosis of the client system's problem.
(4) Examination of alternative routes and goals; establishing goals and intention of action.
(5) Transformation of intentions into actual change efforts.
(6) Generalisation and stabilisation of change.
(7) Achievement of a terminal relationship.[8]

Reflecting the scientific method of investigation and problem solving, most phase models, in one variation or another, account for (1) recognition and engagement with the problem, (2) data collection, (3) diagnosis, (4) intervention and (5) evaluation and termination. While such models are useful in helping the worker think through what needs to be done in a planned change effort, any logical linear sequencing of tasks is an oversimplification of the actual process. The worker may be operating in more than one phase at any one point, and with different types of systems. He may also repeat certain phases at various times. For example, at some point in working with a couple on their marital problems, the worker may decide that the in-laws should be brought into the action system. If the couple is resistant to the idea, the worker may have to reclarify with them his understanding of the nature of the client system's problems and secure a recommitment to the goals and methods of the change effort. If the couple agree, this would then require establishing contact with the in-laws and convincing them of the need to be involved.

Another problem with essentially linear task-accomplishment models is the implication that one phase waits upon the previous one – intervention waits on diagnosis, diagnosis waits on data collection. It is difficult to break out of this pattern of thinking and recognise that all of these activities are occuring throughout the process.

To deal with such problems the concept of process should be viewed in a broader context than that of phase models. 'Process' can be defined as a systematic series of actions directed toward some purpose (or designed to bring about a particular result, end or condition). Process and purpose are thus related concepts. To understand the process in social work practice it is useful to begin with the idea of purpose – what determines the worker's purpose in a given practice situation at any point in time and how these purposes change. While the focus of social work spelt out in the first section of this paper sets the general purpose within which the social worker operates, the interest here is in the more specific purposes and ends toward which the social worker's day-to-day tasks are directed.

The process in social work practice, illustrated in Figure 1, calls for the worker to have a purpose for each activity, as well as for the whole planned change effort. Therefore the same process applies not only to the whole planned change effort but to each activity of the worker within the change effort.

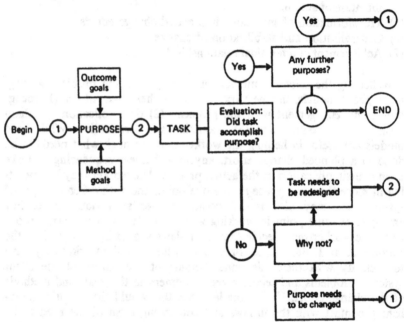

Figure 1   The Process in Social Work Practice

Two main factors help define the worker's purpose: the outcome goals of all systems (client, action, target, change agent) and the method goals of the worker. The worker's purpose is achieved through the accomplishment of specific tasks, as will be discussed later in this section.

Outcome Goals of Systems. An outcome goal is an envisioned end state, a specification of the condition in which we would like to see a situation at the end of a successful planned change effort. Since by our definition the client system is the expected beneficiary of the worker's services, the client's outcome goals should be paramount in determining the worker's purpose. But the outcome goals of the client cannot be viewed in isolation; they must be understood in relation to the outcome goals of all systems involved in a planned change effort. The nature of the relationships (collaborative, bargaining or conflictual) the worker establishes will depend on the congruence of the outcome goals of all those involved. Thus the worker's purpose will be influenced by the outcome goals of the action, target and change agent systems, as well as by those of the client system.

Method Goals of the Worker. While outcome goals refer to the condition in which we would like to see a situation at the end of a successful planned change effort, method goals refer to what must be done in order to bring about this condition. The formation of an action system, the negotiation of a contract with a client, the collection of data about a problem, the conversion of a target system into a client system and the development of adequate decision-making procedures in a committee are examples of method goals. Thus method goals are not sought as ends in themselves but as means to further the achievement of outcome goals.

A key issue is what determines which method goal or goals the worker will pursue. This issue will be considered from the perspectives of points in the planned change process and system maintenance requirements.

Three successive points can be identified which can act as guideposts for the worker in assessing where he is and what method goals he should pursue with respect to each of the four basic systems with which he is working. These points are contact, contract and termination. The social worker will always be working towards one of these points with any given system.

Contact is the initial engagement of a worker and an actual or potential client, action or target system. When a potential client approaches a worker for help with a particular problem, the change effort begins at this point for the worker, although the potential client may have done a lot of thinking about and planning for the initial contact. In cases where the worker 'reaches out' or initiates contact with a potential client, action or target system, careful preparation by the worker for the initial encounter is necessary in order to maximise his effectiveness in influencing them to become a part of the change effort. Indeed, a worker who is new to a community may spend weeks or months studying it and identifying a variety of potential client, action and target systems before establishing any contact related to a specific change effort.

The working agreement or *contract* that must be established by the worker with the client system can be referred to as the primary contract. In addition, the worker will need to come to working agreements with others related to the change effort (action, target and change agent systems). These agreements are secondary contracts.

To some extent the evolution of the contract is a continuing process, as it may be frequently renegotiated. But at some point the worker needs to establish at least a temporary work agreement which defines the nature of his relationship with other persons, the goals and methods of the change effort and the responsibilities of each party. The terms of a contract, as well as commitment to it, may be implicit or explicit.

After a contract is established, the worker will be moving toward the end point in the process, *termination*. The amount of time he spends reaching the goals of the change process will of course vary a great deal from one situation to another, depending on the complexity of the goals and the difficulties encountered along the way. For example, consider a social worker in a hospital who is helping a family cope with the crisis caused by the illness of the mother. Within a week the worker may have arranged for homemaker and after-care services, provided some needed psychological support for the family and, having helped them through the crisis, terminated his relationship with them. As chairman of a committee to improve the co-ordination of hospital services with other community agencies, this same worker may spend a year before reaching that goal and termination. Since members may be added to and dropped from the various systems throughout a given change process, the worker may reach the termination point with different people at different times in the overall process.

In addition to these guideposts, the social worker must be aware of system maintenance requirements. An action system, like any social system, has two major concerns – to achieve specific outcome goals, and to maintain itself as a well-functioning unit. Social systems theory refers to this dual focus as goal achievement and system maintenance. Therefore the method goals of the worker can also be viewed from the perspective of the system needs of the various action systems he forms and works with.

It is important for the worker to keep the action systems functioning smoothly so they can serve as vehicles for the planned change effort. Each action system is an entity in itself and may develop problems which hinder its ability to perform tasks and achieve goals. Problems such as apathy, inability to make decisions, poor communication, conflict or power struggles may arise whether the action system is a community task group, a treatment group, a family or a one-to-one relationship. In any action system the worker must co-ordinate the efforts of different persons and maintain communications. The larger and more complicated the action system, the more time and energy the worker will have to put into system maintenance activities. The worker must not only deal with these problems when they arise but try to form the action system in a way that will minimise their occurrence.

Some of the method goals the worker focuses on are dictated by the needs of these systems, and at different points in their development action systems may pose different problems. Accordingly, the method goals related to action systems will change through time.

From Purpose to Task. After the purposes toward which the process of social work is directed have been determined, the next step is the translation of these purposes into specific tasks that must be accomplished in order to achieve them. The designing and carrying out of these tasks is the heart of practice.[9]

The worker draws on two main sources in linking purposes to tasks. The first is his general knowledge of practice skills. For example, if the worker's purpose is to gather information about a given problem, he will draw on his proficiency in designing and using data collection techniques and his knowledge of which one is most appropriate for collecting the needed data. The task designed to gather needed information may range from an interview at a client's home, to observation of family interaction in a laboratory setting, to a walk around a neighbourhood.

Often a task will be designed with more than one purpose in mind. For example, consider a mother who has come to a mental health centre because of the excessive acting-out behaviour of her 6-year-old child. The mother wants the staff to help the child with his problem. After the initial interview the worker may design a data collection task which requires the mother to record the frequency of certain behaviours of the child at home. In designing this task the worker might have two purposes in mind: to collect more data about the behaviour of the child and to get the mother to see that she will have to take an active part in the treatment process.

A second source the worker draws on in linking purpose to task is his knowledge of theories of behaviour and the dynamics of interactions of individuals, families, groups, organisations and communities. For example, suppose in a given case the worker's purpose is to help alleviate the client's feelings of depression. In order to do this, he must operate on some assumptions about what causes and maintains such behaviour and what can be done to change it. If the worker subscribes to a psychodynamic theory that depression is a result of anger turned inward, he might design a task which involves helping the client express his feelings of anger. Another worker, working from a learning theory perspective, may view the depressive behaviour as a learned response and design a task which involves the reinforcement of non-depressive behaviour. Similarly, workers may have different views on what is causing and maintaining a community problem and what should be done about it.

Since human behaviour and the functioning of social systems are complex topics, any one theory cannot be expected to be adequate for all situations. Further, while some theories offer competing explanations, many are complementary, offering different perspectives on the same situation. Ideally the worker will be familiar with several approaches and pick the one most suitable for his purposes.

The worker may design tasks which (1) he performs himself, (2) the client or others involved in the change effort perform themselves or (3) the worker performs jointly with others. Once a task is completed, the final part of the process is evaluating the extent to which it has accomplished its given purpose. The importance of clarity and specificity in purpose is underscored here. If the worker's purpose is not clear, it will be difficult to tell if and when his purpose has been accomplished. If a given task has failed to accomplish a purpose, or only accomplished it in part, the worker must decide if the task is not appropriate and needs to be redesigned or if he should re-examine his purpose. If a given purpose has been achieved, the process repeats itself until all remaining purposes have been accomplished.

Values
A key concept which needs to be dealt with in any description of practice is that of values. The *primary* values of social work might be stated as follows:

(1) Society has an obligation to ensure that people have access to the resources, services and opportunities they need to meet various life tasks, alleviate distress and realise their aspirations and values.
(2) In providing societal resources, the dignity and individuality of people should be respected.

Value issues permeate all social work practice – the kinds of relationships which are formed, the way situations get defined as problems, the goals for change which get established, and the means employed to reach these goals. One of the reasons that value issues affect all aspects of practice is that ethical ambiguities are inherently built into any change agent role.[10]

To begin with, the reliance on planned change itself ultimately rests on a number of value assumptions: man should not passively accept his conditions but actively intervene to change them; man should make rational use of valid knowledge; man should be future oriented and plan ahead; and so forth. Though the social worker can point to empirical demonstrations of the effects of his planned change efforts to support his faith in the process, he must nonetheless accept the sobering fact that he cannot say with certainty that the world will be better off because of his efforts. Neither can he state with conviction that a given situation might not be worsened rather than improved by his intervention.

In addition to a belief in planned change itself, most social workers subscribe to a set of values governing their working relationships. These are instrumental values such as openness, honesty and collaboration. The change agent may find himself in the position of helping others who either do not share these same values or do not hold them to the same degree. In fact, the worker might diagnose the problems of the client, be it an individual, a family or an organisation, as stemming from the fact that the client is operating on values in conflict with the worker's own instrumental values. For example, the leader of a community organisation may be running the organisation in a very autocratic manner and neglecting to consult the members on important matters or to share enough information with them. As a result the membership may become very apathetic and fail to develop a high commitment to the organisation.

Not only will the practitioner often hold different instrumental values from the client and act upon his own values (impose them) in his relationships with the client, but his very effectiveness depends on his doing so.[11]

Another factor contributing to the ethical ambiguities of practice is that despite any attempts by the worker to maintain a morally neutral stance, the client can still regard the practitioner as a moral agent. There are, in fact, a number of studies which show that psycho-therapists can and do influence client values.[12]

Discussions in the social work literature of the 'limits' of client self-determination[13] point to another set of factors which puts the social worker in a position of interjecting his own values into the planned change process. Though the worker may ideally see his mission as helping people to do what they want, this ideal becomes difficult to apply absolutely in practice. For one thing, the client himself may not be sure about what he wants and indeed may be seeking help in making a decision. The unwed pregnant teenager may be ambivalent about keeping her baby, or the president of a neighbourhood organisation may be unsure about the advisability of merging his organisation with another group in the area. In helping people explore their problems, it is likely that the worker will personally favour one decision or alternative over another. This makes it difficult for the worker not to influence the client's choice by the emphasis he places on different alternatives, the way he presents them or the information he provides.

Even this brief discussion of the concept of the client's self-determination can point to the underlying ethical problem. Social work regards self-determination as a client 'right', but the worker is called upon to decide whether to 'grant' this right to the client and, if so, to what extent. It is a contradiction for the worker to be put in this position. If the worker is able to deny the client's right of self-determination, then it really doesn't, in fact, exist. This is another expression of the value dilemma inherent in the social work role.

How can the change agent meet his responsibility for mitigating the manipulative effects of the planned change process?[14] A first step in coping with the value question is the recognition of its existence, but such a self-awareness is difficult to attain. Ethical questions are ambiguous and make us feel uncomfortable – we like to avoid them. It is also easy to pay lip service to a lofty set of values from a textbook and feel we are meeting our responsibilities in this manner. But abstract values such as client self-determination not only are difficult to use as guides in everyday practice but can be harmful if they lull us into a false sense of complacency.

Self-awareness in and of itself, however, is not enough unless it is put to use in the service of the client. One way the worker can do this is to 'label' his values for the client and allow the client to 'talk back' in a sort of mutual influence situation.

In addition to recognising and limiting the manipulative aspects of the situation, it is important to build into the change process itself procedures that will provide protection and resistance against behaviour manipulation. The situation should be structured in such a way that the client will be encouraged to explore his own values and to relate alternative actions to his own value system. At the same time, the social worker must keep to a minimum the direct and indirect constraints he exercises.

Finally, it is important to go beyond providing clients with protection against manipulation that would encroach on their freedom of choice. The actual *enhancement* of freedom of choice should, ideally, be one of the positive goals of any influence attempt. The worker's professional skills should be used to provide the client with experiences that enhance his ability to choose, and thus to maximise, his own values.

Though these guidelines on coping with the ethical dilemma inherent in the social work role may help, no dilemma yields to a simple or final solution. Armed with self-awareness of values and the knowledge and skills of his profession, the worker is faced with the constant task of maintaining a balance between flexibility and integrity. Flexibility is an essential trait because there must be a mutual accommodation between the expectations of the worker and client in the establishment of an effective relationship. The worker's integrity, however, establishes the boundaries of his flexibility. In establishing such boundaries we will need to identify a personal set of 'bedrock' values. These bedrock values should assure that the worker never loses sight of the mission of his profession – to serve in the best interests of the client. They can also help contain the anxiety which may arise as he experiences the value dilemmas inherent in the change agent role.

PRACTICE SKILLS

We have identified eight essential practice skills which a social worker utilises in performing tasks to carry out the functions of social work.

The worker employs these skills throughout the planned change process with different size and type of systems. We will describe these skills briefly.[15]

Assessing Problems

Throughout the planned change process the worker continually assesses situations and makes decisions about what needs to be done and how to do it. The purpose of the worker's problem assessment is to help him understand and individualise the situation he is dealing with and to identify and analyse the relevant factors in a particular situation. The problem assessment is never an end in itself. Its purpose is not to classify, categorise or assign diagnostic labels to a person or situation. Rather, the decisions about the future course of the planned change effort are the products of the assessment process.

When the worker makes a decision he is in effect making a choice between two or more available alternatives, be it alternative goals, tasks or courses of action. The problem assessment should help identify these alternatives and provide a basis for selection among them.

Many factors enter into the worker's problem assessment. Though the format will vary from one work setting to another, any problem assessment will include the following:

(1) Identifying and stating the problem – focusing on three elements that comprise any problem: the behaviours or social condition in question, the people who are evaluating it and the reasons for their evaluations. We stress that in assessing problems the worker should not view the problem as the property of a given person or persons, but as characteristic of their interactions.
(2) Analysing the dynamics of the social situation – developing an understanding of how all the systems connected to the situation are operating to produce or maintain behaviours or social conditions.
(3) Establishing goals and targets – including consideration of sub-goals, feasibility and priorities.
(4) Determining tasks and strategies – developing an intervention plan specifying who is to do what in what order and at what point in time.
(5) Stabilising the change effort – anticipating what new problems might arise as a result of the planned change effort and what needs to be done to see that change is maintained once it is achieved.

Collecting Data

Many problems confronting the social worker will require data collection on and from a variety of systems. Data collection techniques can be divided into three major categories:

(1) Questioning
   A. Direct verbal questioning (individual and group interviewing)
   B. Direct written questioning (application forms, survey question-
      naire)
   C. Projective and other indirect verbal and written techniques (role
      playing, sentence completion tasks)
(2) Observing
   A. Observing behaviour and social interaction
   B. Observing inanimate objects
(3) Using Existing Written Materials
   A. Material intended for use by social workers (e.g. case records,
      minutes of committee meetings)
   B. 'Raw' material not originally intended for use by social workers
      (e.g. newspaper stories, letters)
   C. Systematically organised data (e.g. population census statistics,
      budgets of agencies)

While a wide array of data collection techniques is available to a social worker, in any given situation he may not have much choice as to which techniques to use. When possible, planned use of appropriate techniques should yield the maximum amount of valid data. The use of more than one mode of data collection should be considered whenever possible. Certain techniques are best for certain kinds of data, but each technique has its own advantages and disadvantages. The disadvantages of any single technique can be minimised only if it is used in combination with other techniques.

The worker's data is the raw material for his problem assessment. However, because of the selectivity which must go into data collection (there is no way to collect all possible information about a given person or situation), it is all too easy for the worker to collect data to support preconceived assessments and decisions. Thus the social worker faces a dilemma in the data collection process. On the one hand, he must be selective in how he collects his data and approach the process with some orientation and assumptions to guide his effort. On the other hand, his orientation and assumptions can operate to bias and distort the data collection process to such an extent that all objectivity is lost. The worker must keep flexible enough to disregard his assumptions when they are not substantiated by the data, instead of building rigid frameworks which effectively filter out any data not supporting his original assumptions.

Making Initial Contact
Contact is the initial engagement or coming together of a worker and a potential or actual client, action or target system. The first encounter

may occur when the system seeks out the worker on its own or through a referral by a third party. Often a worker himself will reach out and make the initial contact. Throughout any change process, the social worker will ordinarily make initial contact with several people. As a change effort unfolds, contact will have to be established with potential members of an action system, additional potential clients and target systems.

When the social worker is initiating contact with potential client, action or target systems, all parties may be ambivalent about beginning a change effort. In order to engage people in change efforts, the social worker will need to analyse their perception of the *benefits* they believe will accrue to them from the change effort and what they believe the change effort will *cost* them. The worker can use his analysis of the other systems' perceptions of costs and benefits to plan a strategy for contact that will stimulate positive motivations and reduce or minimise resistance forces.

Several forces that may lead individuals, groups, organisations and communities to resist change efforts can be identified. These are (1) reluctance to accept help, (2) fear of loss of position or resources, (3) belief that change is impossible, (4) reluctance to devote time, (5) practical barriers to participation and (6) uncertainty.

On the other hand, several forces may motivate people to become involved in change efforts. These are (1) willingness to accept help, (2) desire to gain position or resources, (3) belief that change is possible, (4) relief from discomfort, (5) response to constraints, and (6) altruism.

When a worker is reaching out to another system, his first task is to decide what part or parts of the system to contact to begin the change effort. He may be reaching out to a multiple-person system (family, neighbourhood group, another community agency or institution) or trying to make contact with other systems connected to an ongoing change effort. If the worker is proposing a change that will have an impact on the functioning of the entire system, he can expect to find resistance and motivating forces operating with the many sub-parts of the system. He will want to make his contacts with those parts that can exert influence within the entire system to reduce resistance and enhance motivations for change.

The social worker may choose a contact strategy from a variety of methods. The social worker may: directly approach another system, ask someone with high status or someone whom the target system has learned to trust to make the initial contact, use contact people who themselves are current or recent members of the target population (drug addicts, ex-convicts, poor people), use a special facility that suits the life style of the target population for first contacts (teenage drop-in centre, neighbourhood store front), locate themselves where people are when they need help (unemployment offices, jails) or use the mass media.

Negotiating Contracts

Once the social worker and another system make contact, his major method goal is to influence people in the other system to become involved in the change effort. His first step in accomplishing this goal is to negotiate a contract with them.

When social workers and other systems begin to work together, all parties bring to the encounter some initial expectations about how they and the other should or will act, and what should or will happen. As people begin to interact with one another, their initial expectations may be modified. Patterns or norms of behaviour become established. Understanding develops between the parties about the rules of the game and what they have decided to do (or not do) together. These understandings result in formal or informal working agreements.

We will refer to these working agreements as contracts. We use the term to call attention to the existence of such working agreements between parties in a change effort, whether or not the social worker and the other systems explicitly recognise them. The term also emphasises the contractual nature of the relationships, in which both parties have obligations to fulfil. Thus a contract is not something that the worker imposes on another system. Rather it is the deliberate and conscious articulation and shaping of the informal working agreements that are inherent in all relationships into a form that will facilitate the planned change process.

The basic factors to be agreed upon in contracts between social workers and other systems (change agent, client, action and target) are:

(1) Major goals of the parties.
(2) Tasks to be performed by each party to achieve the goals.
(3) Operating procedures for the change process.

An essential element of each of these factors is a clear delineation of the responsibility of each party for meeting the terms of the contract.

In negotiating a contract with another system, the social worker uses divers techniques to involve other people and secure a mutually acceptable working agreement. In practice he combines many of these techniques into an overall strategy, but some are particularly helpful for specific purposes, such as (1) establishing an initial relationship with another system, (2) identifying the purpose of the contract, (3) clarifying contract terms and (4) identifying disagreements with the other system. The worker may have to deal directly with the resistances of other systems in order to reach agreement on a contract. He can use a variety of techniques to overcome resistance, including involving other systems, acknowledging resistance, upsetting equilibrium to create a temporary crisis, providing hope, establishing short-term or trial goals, getting help from other people and using groups for intake.

The contract between the worker and other systems may be negotiated in one meeting or the negotiation may last for several sessions. Once a contract is negotiated, it does not remain static but can be formally or informally renegotiated several times in a change effort.

Forming Action Systems

The action system is composed of the social worker and the people he works with to accomplish tasks and achieve method and outcome goals. In any one change effort, the worker may form many different action systems to collect data, assess the problem, make an initial contact, negotiate a contract or influence the major targets to help achieve the outcome goal.

The action system is the medium through which the worker influences the targets of change. Its effectiveness can be enhanced by careful planning in its formation and operation. The social worker forming action systems must operate within the constraints of three major characteristics of action systems: size, composition and operating procedures.

Size. In planning any change effort the social worker must determine what size action systems will be most effective to achieve his purposes and influence the targets. The worker's decision on the most effective and efficient size action system to use is influenced by two major factors: the purpose he hopes to achieve and the characteristics of the target. The most effective size action system to be established for the achievement of a particular purpose could be either a one-to-one or a group action system. Often use can also be made of existing action systems. However, the worker's choice of a one-to-one or group action system also may be determined by his need to gain the participation of the target in the change effort. His choice is also predetermined if the target will agree to a proposal or suggestion of the worker only in either a one-to-one or group action system.

Composition. The worker must choose, perhaps from a number of candidates, the particular people to include in a specific action system. He will be concerned with putting together the best mix of people who will contribute to and gain from the action system. The worker must select people who will help the action system itself function smoothly. At the same time he must select those who will help each other learn something from action system membership that can be transferred to other situations and those who will perform tasks outside the action system to help it achieve its purpose. In considering people who can contribute to both the internal functioning and the external purpose and tasks of the action system, the worker is guided in his selection by two kinds of attributes of potential action system members – descriptive and behavioural. A descriptive attribute describes a person in a position (teenager, parent of a mentally retarded child, president of a school board, a black neighbourhood resident). A behavioural attribute refers to the way a person acts in a position (a teenager who plays alone, a parent who is a strict disciplinarian, a school board president who acts as a compromiser, a neighbourhood resident who speaks up at meetings). The worker can influence both the internal functioning and the accomplishment of external tasks and purposes of an action system by selecting members with appropriate descriptive and behavioural attributes.

Operating Procedures. Social workers can influence the functioning of an action system by the use of time, by planning for the setting or place of interaction and by establishing norms or rules for interaction and decision making. These factors operate in all systems whether they are one-to-one or group action systems.

Maintaining and Co-ordinating Action Systems

An action system becomes a social entity after it has been put together by a worker and members begin to interact. In analysing problems that arise in the internal functioning of the system and threaten the achievement of its purposes, the worker views the action system both from a developmental and a social system perspective.

The developmental perspective is concerned with the history of the interactions of the members of the action system, considering where the relationships among members are now in reference to where they have been and how they might develop in future. The social system perspective focuses on the internal functioning of the system at one moment in time.

At any one stage in the development of an action system, problems may arise that will prevent the members from accomplishing the tasks at that stage and from moving on through the stages of development to achieve its purpose. Problems in the functioning of action systems can result from (1) role distribution, (2) communications, (3) interpersonal relationships, (4) the distribution of power, (5) conflicting loyalties, (6) conflicting values and attitudes or (7) the nature of the purpose.

In order to resolve the various types of problems that arise in the action systems, the social worker must first diagnose the problem and then decide which of several techniques he will employ to deal with it.

The worker might (1) assume different roles, (2) change the operating procedures, (3) regulate the use of programme and activities, (4) change the membership of the action system or (5) assist members to diagnose their problems.

Problems may arise not only between members of a single action system but between people in different action systems. As has been noted, the worker can form a number of action systems to deal with a particular problem. Unless the efforts of these action systems are co-ordinated, the systems may be working at cross-purposes, so that they hinder rather than aid the worker and his clients in achieving their goals.

Exercising Influence
The exercise of influence underlies most of the interaction activities of the social worker as he carries out his tasks in a planned change effort. In collecting data in an interview, the worker will try to create a climate conducive to open discussion. In negotiating a contract, he will try to heighten the other person's motivation to participate in the change effort. When forming a task group, he may try to convince a certain person to serve as chairman. The social worker who understands the dynamics of influence processes will be able to harness and use them in conscious ways to facilitate the achievement of outcome and method goals.

Broadly speaking, the term 'influence' can be defined as affecting the condition or development of a person or system. The exercise of influence is usually a two-way transactional process. Its use depends both on the target's perception of the person attempting to exert influence and on the target's attitude toward being influenced. It is also a two-way process, in the sense that the worker himself will often become a target of other people's influence attempts.

When the exercise of influence in social work is carefully examined, it is always possible to identify some base of influence the worker brings to bear in order to affect a situation. These bases of influence include (1) knowledge and expertness, (2) material resources and services, (3) legitimate authority, (4) status and reputation, (5) charisma and personal attractiveness, (6) control over the flow of information and (7) established relationships. The social worker may directly control or possess any of these resources himself, or he may have access to people who can bring them to bear in a situation.

In exercising influence a change agent must not only control a base of influence but must be able to bring it to bear on a target system. Four major means of influence (or influence processes) used by social workers to change a target system's behaviour, attitudes and beliefs are: (1) inducement, (2) persuasion, (3) use of relationship and (4) use of environment. The social worker can use some combination of these means of influence to achieve method and outcome goals in performing the various functions of social work practice.

Several issues can arise in the social worker's use of the different means of influence. These can involve combination of the means of influences, the limitations of influence resources, the communication of influence, the cost of exercising influence and value implications of the use of influence.

Terminating the Change Effort

Termination is not just some point reached at the end of the planned change effort, but an integral part of the whole process which the worker carefully prepares for and helps bring about. Skills in terminating a planned change effort and disengaging from relationships are as necessary as skills in initiating the effort and engaging people in it. The way the process is brought to an end can affect the success of the whole change effort and future relationships between the worker and members of the client, action and target systems.

The groundwork for termination is laid throughout the planned change process. Time limits established in the beginning provide a target date to work toward and against which progress can be measured. The formulation of clear and specific outcome goals makes it easier to assess the extent to which they have been realised. In addition to this groundwork, there are specific things the worker must do near the end of the planned change effort to help bring it to a successful conclusion. These include (1) evaluation of the change effort, (2) disengaging from relationships and (3) stabilisation of the change effort.

Evaluation should be a continuing activity throughout the planned change process. After each task has been completed, the worker must determine if it has accomplished its purpose and decide if the methods or goals of the change effort should be re-adjusted or redefined. From time to time the worker and client or action systems may engage in a broader review and assessment of the progress being made, particularly if no time limits have been established. Reaching some impasse or getting 'bogged down' should signal the need to take stock and reassess what is being done. While the evaluation at the end of the process is more comprehensive, it should be a continuation of the evaluative activity throughout the planned change process.

When disengaging from relationships, the worker must understand the dynamics of endings and be prepared to cope with a variety of reactions to it. The prospects of termination may be accompanied by ambivalent feelings by all parties to a change effort, particularly if participation in an action system has been a rewarding experience.

The third major task the worker must be concerned with at the time of termination is the stabilisation and generalisation of the change effort.

He needs to assess the steps which must be taken to make sure that the positive changes and gains will be maintained after he is no longer involved.

SUMMARY AND CONCLUSION

As indicated in the introduction, our model of social work practice was developed in response to the limitations we saw in conceptualising social work according to the traditional three divisions of casework, group work and community organisation. By way of concluding this chapter we wish to note a number of characteristics of our model we believe have helped to correct those limitations.

First, our model should avoid conceptualising social work practice in such dichotomous terms as person/environment, clinical practice/social action and microsystems/macrosystems. We believe the strength of the profession lies in recognising and working with the connections between these elements.

Secondly, our model accounts for the fact that the worker has tasks to perform and relationships to maintain with a variety of people in any planned change effort. Work with people other than the client is seen as deliberate and purposeful activity. The model focuses on the relationship of these people to the planned change effort and in skills in working with them as well as the client.

Thirdly, the worker will often have to work with and through many different sizes and types of systems (one-to-one relationships, families, community groups) in helping a client. The methods of practice suggested by the model are not to be tied to any one size of system. The appropriate size and type of system or systems to work through depends on the nature of the task at hand.

Fourthly, the model is not based on any one substantive theoretical orientation, such as learning theory, ego psychology, communication theory or conflict resolution, but allows for the selective incorporation of such theoretical orientations in working with specific situations. The social work model for practice is clearly differentiated from any substantive theoretical orientations being utilised. In many practice models the two become so intertwined that the theoretical orientation appears to dictate the purpose of the social worker's practice. A social work frame of reference, derived from a clear notion of the function and purpose of the profession, avoids this problem by serving as the primary guide in analysing and dealing with social situations.

Fifthly, while the model is applicable to analysing social work in a wide variety of situations and settings in which it is practised, it does account for the skills, tasks and activities of the social worker at a very specific level, rather than an abstract one.

Though we have borrowed many useful ideas from existing conceptualisations of practice and adapted them to our model, we want to make it clear that our model does not propose a supramethod of practice that integrates or combines casework, group work and community work. What our model integrates is ways of understanding the nature of social work practice, the role of the social worker and the skills he uses in carrying out his role. It hopefully represents a reformulation of the base of social work practice which gives social work a clear place among the human service professions.

NOTES AND REFERENCES FOR CHAPTER 5

1 Allen Pincus and Anne Minahan, *Social Work Practice: Model and Method* (Itasca, Ill.: Peacock, 1973).
2 For elaboration of the concept of life tasks, see Harriet M. Bartlett, *The Common Base of Social Work Practice*, p. 96.
3 See Pincus and Minahan, *Social Work Practice*, pp. 16–33 for a description of social work tasks and activities.
4 See Felix B. Biestek, *The Casework Relationship* (Chicago: Loyola University Press, 1957); Florence Hollis, *Casework – A Psychological Therapy* (New York: Random House, 1972); Helen Northern, *Social Work with Groups* (New York: Columbia University Press, 1969); Carl R. Rogers, *Freedom to Learn* (Columbus, Ohio: Merrill, 1969) and *On Becoming a Person* (Boston: Houghton Mifflin, 1961).
5 Chris Argyris, 'Explorations in consulting-client relationships', in Warren Bennis, Kenneth Benne and Robert Chin (eds), *The Planning of Change*, 2nd edn (New York: Holt, Rinehart & Winston, 1969), pp. 434–57; Murray Ross, *Community Organization: Theory and Principles* (New York: Harper & Row, 1955).
6 Roland Warren, 'Types of purposive social change at the community level', Brandeis University Papers in Social Welfare, no. 11 (Waltham, Mas., 1965); Harry Specht, 'Disruptive tactics', *Social Work*, vol. XIV, no. 2 (April 1969), pp. 5–15.
7 George A. Brager, 'Advocacy and political behavior', *Social Work*, no. 13 (April 1968), p. 6.
8 Ronald Lippitt, Jeanne Watson and Bruce Westley, *The Dynamics of Planned Change* (New York: Harcourt, Brace & World, 1958), pp. 131–43.
9 For an elaboration of the task concept as central to social work practice, see William J. Reid, 'Target problems, time limits, task structure', *Journal of Education for Social Work*, no. 8 (Spring 1972), pp. 58–68, and Elliot Studt, 'Social work theory and implications for the practice of methods', *Social Work Education Reporter*, no. 16 (June 1968), pp. 22–7.
10 Herbert C. Kelman, 'Manipulation of human behavior: an ethical dilemma for the social scientist', in Bennis, Benne and Chin (eds), *The Planning of Change*, pp. 582–95.
11 Chris Argyris, 'Explorations in consulting-client relationships'.
12 David Rosenthal, 'Changes in some moral values following psychotherapy', *Journal of Consulting Psychology*, no. 19 (November 1955), pp. 431–6.
13 See Saul Bernstein, 'Self-determination: king or citizen in the realm of values?' *Social Work*, no. 5 (January 1960), pp. 3–8; Alan Keith-Lucas, 'A

critique of the principle of client self-determination', *Social Work*, no. 8 (July 1963), pp. 66–71; David Soyer, 'The right to fail', *Social Work*, no. 8 (July 1963), pp. 72–8.

14 Much of the following discussion is based on Kelman, *Manipulation of Human Behavior*.

15 Each of the eight practice skills is discussed in a separate chapter in Pincus and Minahan, *Social Work Practice*.

PART II

CONTENT TO BE INTEGRATED

Conceptions of man as 'an integrated whole' and as a 'system' with a unique integrity interacting with other systems that have their unique integrity are inherently appealing. Interest in general systems theory and ecological approaches abounds in the community and in the professions and sciences. Efforts to understand the ways in which 'everything is related to everything else' are generated, in large part, by a desire to grasp and to exercise greater control over technology and knowledge that has grown in size and complexity to a degree that is beyond people's comprehension.

In Part II we discuss the complex and varied ideas, theories and beliefs that constitute social work practice. The reader will find that, unlike the orderly discussion in the first part, which was about theory in social work, the descriptions of the specifics of practice in the following pages will not be orderly. This is because, we believe, neat and tidy explanations of behaviour can be achieved only at very high levels of generalisation. Of course, neat and tidy high-level generalisations have their use in helping us orient ourselves 'in relation to everything else'. However, after the traveller has located himself in relation to the sun, the moon and the stars, he must attend to the subtle twists and turns of the trail, watch out for protruding branches, take care to avoid that rut and find a place to pitch his tent for the night that will not be too uncomfortable.

Similarly, practitioners who deal with individuals, families and groups on a day-to-day basis develop their major orientations from grander theories. Beyond that, they use a mix of lower-level theory, guesswork and intuition to get the job done. In the following pages we describe these mixes as they have been articulated for casework, group work and community work practice and for practice in residential work.

In Chapter 6, entitled 'Social work in the future: trends and training', Dame Eileen Younghusband describes the enormous pressure of knowledge and tasks that are coming to bear upon social work. Education for practice, she says, is under increasing strain 'as courses struggle to stuff in added knowledge and more varied field work placements without too clear an idea of how much students effectively use in subsequent practice'.

In Chapter 7, Anne Vickery discusses the variety of perspectives on, and theoretical approaches to, social casework. The literature on this mode of intervention is both older and more extensive than other methodological specialisations. Vickery enables us to see how the varying goals and functions of casework are supported by different theoretical views of practice. She draws out the problematic issues with which these variations confront practitioners.

Chapter 8 is a paper by Catherine Papell and Beulah Rothman in which they describe the different models of social group work. In 'Social group work models: possession and heritage', they discuss how the elements of group work practice have been ordered by these models. Development of these models of social group work, Papell and Rothman note, has enriched social work from both a theoretical and practice point of view. In Chapter 9, Nano McCaughan describes the current development of social group work in the United Kingdom.

In 'Community work in the United Kingdom', Chapter 10, David Jones traces the connections among group work, social administration, community development and community work. In Jones's view there is a continuum of social work methods ranging from casework to social administration. Community work, he says, consists of practices concerned with activities involving work with community groups, administration and social planning. In the following chapter, Catherine Briscoe specifies how some of these ideas have entered into the current practice of community work in the United Kingdom.

In the last chapter of Part II, residential work is described by Chris Payne as a social work method that has more that is in common with than is different from community-based social work. He describes the elements and the conditions required to achieve the integration of residential work with other kinds of social work.

Chapter 6

SOCIAL WORK IN THE FUTURE: TRENDS AND TRAINING*

Eileen Younghusband

On a subject so enormous as new interventions in social work and what this means for training all I can do is give you a few scattered thoughts. This is not going to be a finished paper in which you can all sit back and let it flow over your heads: it's going to be a series of issues and problems to think about and carry farther in discussion. Neither you nor I know the answers, but what we all need is to clarify some of the questions, to air some views about which we feel strongly and about which we think this or that ought or ought not to happen.

First of all, then, there's a kind of egg and chicken relationship between training and the day-to-day working policies, resources and their use in different social services or social work departments. It's not possible in any fundamental way for good training to shift the policies of a department but conversely dim-witted policies can't shift without good training of the staff on whom implementation depends. And both are ultimately dependent upon the calibre of those who come forward to train for social work. Thank goodness there's been a great shift in this in my professional lifetime. Indeed social work has become almost a mainstream option amongst students choosing a career.

It's no longer confined to middle-class spinsters who wanted to become caseworkers but didn't want to be promoted to managerial/administrative jobs. Don't think I'm decrying casework or the middle-class spinsters. We're going to be more and more hard put to it to close all the gaps left without the latter's reliable presence, their tendency to stay in the same job and to become known in the district. Nor am I decrying casework. There probably ought to be a good deal more of it, more selectively used, and it certainly ought to be much better than it is at present.

The essence of the point I'm making at the moment is that until

* This paper was presented at the Institute of Continuing Education, New University of Ulster, at its conference on 'New Interventions in Social Work', June 1973. It is printed here with the permission of the author.

recently we have had an extremely constricted view of the whole operation of social services/social work. Our sights were limited, sometimes unrealistic, rather than low, but now there's a revolution going on which has stretched the boundaries of the whole operation. Instead of confining casework to working with and mobilising resources on behalf of individual people under stress, and restricting group work mainly to informal education activities with socially starved young people, we're beginning to see that it's manifestly absurd to try to bring about change in individuals or small groups alone when the job also demands substantial structural change and changes in local people's ability to gain more control over the circumstances of their lives, to feel – and be – more competent, to gain confidence through being respected for real achievement. The effect on Sunderland of their team winning the Cup tie is a recent dramatic example of what achievement and recognition does to people at the end of the line.

Anyway, the general point is a swing from the negative to the positive in our concept of social services. 'It shall be the duty of the local authority to promote welfare in its area', as Section 12 of the Scottish Social Work Act puts it. There are three points here which all relate to training. The first is that this kind of concept implies a much wider range of skills than direct-service casework alone; the second related point is that this wider definition of the nature of social work attracts to it a broader range of candidates for training than those who are attracted to a narrowly conceived type of casework. The third point is that education for social work, and thus the definable profession of social work, has got to discover how to encompass this wider range of social intervention processes at a respectable level of professional practice.

This raises many dilemmas that face us at present. For example, training must not be too badly out of step with what is happening in the field. Effective social intervention entails very much more sophisticated diagnosis and a wider range of available resources than are commonly available at the present time. But students must be able when they qualify to begin to work usefully in existing social services as well as to grow and develop so that they can contribute to the better services, the greater clear-sightedness, the ability to reinforce the constructive forces for social change to which with essential optimism we look forward.

This reminds us that there are three parties to the whole enterprise: the employer and provider of resources, mainly local authorities, the recipients of the services and – in our context – social workers. Each of these may have different views about the nature and dimensions of the task. Local authorities are sometimes progressive, sometimes stick-in-the-mud with little concept of their contribution to social change, of the right of ordinary people to take initiative in deciding priorities. These people themselves may not know about services or use them effectively; moreover their views about human behaviour are often much more moralistic, so far as others are concerned, than are those of social workers trained to ask not 'who is to blame and should be brought to heel' but 'what contributed to this deadlock in human relationships and what needs to shift – and how?' Social workers also sometimes find themselves in conflict with their employing organisation about people's right to protest, to have their grievances put at the forefront of the agenda. The degree of tension this causes is partly related to the kind of leadership given by the chief officers, the extent to which they are professionally competent and unite managerial skills with liberal objectives.

All this related intimately to training. Students ought to confront these issues with the psychological, sociological, economic, political and ethical strands in them; and social work as a profession needs constantly to try to work out guidelines. These guidelines or ethics of professional practice should be based upon analysis of experience and be an essential support for social workers faced by the risk of rigidity, withdrawal or loss of a sense of direction.

I am assuming, then, for the purpose of this discussion, that social work includes a range of relationships and interventions with and on behalf of individuals, families, groups and communities. As they used to say in Bermondsey when I lived in a settlement there: 'That sounds fine if you say it quick enough.' But it's very different in application to practice, and thus to student training. For example, training would be more effective if we had fairly precise 'hard' knowledge about the application of theory to practice which we could help students to learn to apply. But we haven't reached that point yet. Moreover, most of the available knowledge comes from the social and behavioural sciences, which are already top-heavy with patchy knowledge or with tentative hypotheses and with conflicting theories which must be mastered by students within some coherent frame of reference. But social work is the opposite of top-heavy when it comes to the application of relevant concepts to the theory and practice of social work.

Take community work as an example: there's a good deal that is relevant to it in sociology, social psychology, economics and political theory. There's also a rapidly increasing practice of community work. But the thing that comes in the middle is almost non-existent in Britain, that is to say the application of the theory to recorded and tested practice; yet this is necessary to build up a transmissible body of what the Americans call practice theory. A result is that so far it is extremely difficult to give students very much more than practice which lacks transmissible skills about the essentials and theory which, however stimulating, often only seems applicable by the high-ups in Kingdom Come.

The situation is not at quite so early a stage of development so far as casework is concerned. This is because about twenty-five years ago we began to lower our resistances enough to profit from American experience and to let it grow and change when we applied it to our own situation. Of course this was easier in some ways because the dynamic psychology on which casework was largely based had itself been evolved by practitioners, whereas sociologists were researchers and theoreticians who had only recently begun to think it could be respectable to apply knowledge to practice. In saying this I'm not engaging in any of the 'better' or 'worse', 'goodies' and 'baddies' controversies. It's wholly a good thing if we are broadening our perceptions of dynamic psychology and are now also able to take account of the equally valid cultural, social perspective in human behaviour.

Casework with individuals and families and community work in group and inter-group situations or in inter-agency or social planning contexts, are, I would argue, two ends of a continuum. Once more, it's the thing in between that's neglected. In this context I mean work with groups. Casework has had the limelight for a number of years. Community work has suddenly generated vitality, has begun to burgeon in both employment and training. But group work remains, as it has been for years, essentially neglected in Britain. I say this recognising ventures with un-attached youth, in mental hospitals, in prisons; together with group discussion by caseworkers with, for example, single parents, would-be adopters or prisoners' wives. I know also that in many professional trainings for social work there are now short courses in group dynamics or the students have more or less searing or illuminating experiences in 'T' groups.

Obviously group work could be in some respects a conciliator in all the conflicts between casework and community work because both of them by the very nature of the task and their employment in social agencies are working constantly in group and inter-group situations. Moreover, in our newly widening perceptions we are beginning to see that the 'social care' function in residential situations like children's homes or for old or handicapped or delinquent or deviant people is a very complex form of social work with groups and individuals in what ought to be a therapeutic community rather than a dead end or a dustbin.

To come back once more to the point from which I keep on straying, how much of this can be encompassed in any one type of training for social work? And, of course, how much of it is social work exclusively, not anything else? Let's deal with the second point first and just to give you a personal view I think that casework in the form of a systematic helping relationship with individuals under stress, plus making arrangements and combining public or voluntary social resources plus local good will in ways relevant to an individual situation is uniquely itself as casework, even though to some extent it overlaps with clinical psychology and with some psychiatry. Is social group work uniquely itself even though it overlaps with informal education and with group psychotherapy? And what about the question mark that hangs over community work? This really *is* a question mark at the present time. There are some community workers who wouldn't want to be seen dead in the ditch with social workers. In their view community work is an essentially egalitarian process with normal people, aimed at helping them to reach and carry out their own decisions and to act as their advocates in relation to the power structure, whereas casework is a non-egalitarian process carried on by social workers who think they are professionals but who don't understand their clients' culture or point of view, are largely concerned with what they call unconscious motivation in which they use their skills to induce clients to conform to middle-class values, i.e. to toe the line that the establishment decides. All social work is practised along another continuum, one which ranges from social change/reform to social control. Some would deny that this *is* a continuum rather than two irreconcilable polar opposites. At any rate, a basic issue for social work practice and education is how far the boundaries stretch at either end.

New developments in community work and in training for it are forcing into the centre these fundamental questions about social values, about the relations between the individual and the state, about the uses and abuses of community action. Most students in social work courses go through a stage when they come sharp up against the question of whether their new understanding of human motivation will be used in social agencies to manoeuvre people into conformity. They also go through a stage when the demand on them to become more aware of themselves and others, to face their own prejudices and to stretch their imagination, seems like brain-washing. Personally I think students must experience these demands on their minds and their emotions, if they are to feel the impact, the complexity, of social values of conflicting demands, and to learn to tolerate uncertainty in their professional practice.

This is also part of the case for training. The untrained have little but their own experience from which to learn, they may find it difficult to transfer whatever they have learned from one situation to another and they have not got the support of accepted but, let us hope, improving standards of professional practice, the acceptance of a code that reinforces and supports personal integrity. As I've said in another context, this latter is extremely important in situations where the worker may face enormous pressures to take sides, to use undue influence, to lose his sense of direction.

In all I've said I have implied that substantial field practice under competent field teachers is a necessary part of all training for social work. This seems to me crucial. There is no other way so far discovered to close the gap between knowledge and the ability to use it in practice. I had a good demonstration of this recently when I was giving a driving lesson to a boy who knew a great deal about the insides of cars – about which I know nothing – but had no experience of actually driving one. The lesson ended dramatically in the ditch and thus reinforced all my prejudices about the difference between knowledge in itself and skill in its application. Of course it also demonstrated the inadequacy of my own teaching skills.

This leads into one of the biggest problems facing social work education at present. If we accept that the practice of social work includes relationships with individuals, groups and communities and sophisticated use of both formal and indigenous resources, then how much of all this can be included at the basic training stage or must be added selectively later? Is it more productive to train students for fairly narrow specialisation but on principles that are essentially generic, or should they be introduced to a wider range or to the whole range of social work? If the latter, can they achieve any solid basis for generic practice with individuals, groups and communities? Is there sufficient common ground between the three to make this possible? Or would the attempt result in a general superficiality in which they do not even begin to know enough, or to have a solid working basis? If, alternatively, they are to put the emphasis on either casework – direct service – or community work at different levels, is there a sufficient common body of knowledge between these so that students leave feeling that they belong to one profession rather than having diverged beyond common understanding and respect? In any event, where does group work come in? As I said earlier, understanding of the dynamics of the group is essential to both casework and community work, but is it used too differently in small therapeutic groups and in the inter-group situations of community work for there to be a sufficient common base? And in any event has group work no validity in its own right? How will it develop within itself if it is simply an adjunct to other forms of practice?

This problem is becoming more and more pressing as courses struggle to stuff in added knowledge and more varied fieldwork placements without too clear an idea of how much students effectively use in subsequent practice. It seems pretty clear that there's got to be longer and better training for some people. But what and when? Is it more productive to undergo a wide-ranging and thus longer basic training or a narrower one followed by opportunities for more diversified advanced training for some people as they go up the professional ladder? Would this advanced training include much more sophistication in applying diagnostic skill to situations and in the use of social intervention strategies? What about 'conversion' courses for people who want to step sideways, for example from casework to community work or residential care to fieldwork – or vice versa? Is the time past when we thought that ideally a social services department should be staffed by professionally qualified social workers? At present we think of welfare assistants and volunteers as important in their own right rather than as not quite respectable stop-gaps. But they need on-the-job training and constant support if they are to be adequately used. Who is to train the trainers here and elsewhere?

Then there's the whole question of how to close the gaps between employment and training. As a major example, most real learning is learning on the job. Does the whole current concept of continuous education entail systematic staff development as well as periodic chances of going away for short courses? And what are the criteria for evaluating the effectiveness of this? The aim presumably is to give sufficient support and chances for development to social workers so that they both stay on the job and do it more effectively, i.e. that both they and their employing authorities respond more accurately to the changing nature of the task.

These are just a few of the issues facing social work education at the present time. You'll be well aware of all I've left out and all the complexities I've not faced. But it's healthy for us to look at these issues rather than ignoring or feeling defeated by them.

Chapter 7

SOCIAL CASEWORK

Anne Vickery

'A great temptation, yielded to more often than resisted, leads each generation to enhance its own self-esteem by emphasising the short-comings of its predecessors....'

Florence Hollis, 'Contemporary issues for caseworkers', *Smith College Studies in Social Work*, vol. XXX, no. 2 (1960)

INTRODUCTION

On several grounds it has become fashionable to castigate social case-work. It is thought to be too much concerned with changing the personal behaviour of clients and too little concerned with changing their environment. Allegedly it relies too exclusively on psychoanalytic theory and fails to use knowledge derived from experimental psychology, small group theory and the insights of sociological and political theory.

But many criticisms of social casework are based on its goals and theoretical orientations as derived from social casework literature. Fewer are based on observations of actual casework practice. Nevertheless, there are a number of evaluative studies that do assess the kinds of goals that may be realistic for casework to pursue and which suggest certain ingredients that might be crucial to their achievement.[1]

We have discussed some of the evaluations of casework in the section on social trends (Chapter 1). Our purpose here is to consider what it is that distinguishes casework from other forms of social work. In doing so it will be possible to touch on only a few of the conceptual issues and historical events that have influenced social casework in recent decades. Readers who desire a more detailed account of the various conceptualisations and comparative analyses of different casework approaches should refer to the original sources.[2]

THE GOALS OF SOCIAL CASEWORK

Casework goals vary considerably in practice. Goldstein[3] provides a framework for examining types of goals which, though addressed to social work practice as a whole, greatly illuminates discussion about the ends and means of casework, and the appropriate cut-off point for the caseworker's efforts. He distinguishes five types of social work goals, three of which are concerned with aspects of environmental change, and the other two with more personally focused goals. The three concerned with aspects of environmental change are: (1) *concrete change*, such as housing and income; (2) *structural change*, such as modification of a social system; (3) change in *current reality*, referring to immediate 'first-aid' work. The more personally focused goals are: (4) *'foresight' goals*, by which Goldstein means the identification of what the client wishes to achieve; and (5) *'vitalistic' goals*, by which he means nurturing the client's capacity for personal growth. These last two personally focused goals have often been stated as comprising *the* aim of casework, with the environmental goals being viewed as a means to that end.

To clarify the ends and means of social work practice Goldstein makes three further distinctions among goals: he defines goals that are 'optimal' (i.e. those that are ultimate desired ends), goals that are 'interim' (i.e. those that are significant milestones toward desired ends) and goals that are 'facilitative' (i.e. those that make it possible to begin the process of goal achievement). These last three goals identify stages in the social work process; they cut across and form a matrix with the first-mentioned set of goals, any one of which can be viewed as optimal, interim or facilitative. For example, one client may view his placement in a hostel (i.e. a concrete goal) as an optimal goal; another may consider it to be an interim goal in a process of rehabilitation from the hospital to achieving independence in the community; another may view it as a facilitative goal, providing a roof over his head and a chance to start working on problems.

Many of the criticisms of casework arise from a tendency in the casework literature to describe optimal goals in vague and ambitious terms such as, 'to help people realise their potential'. In these instances it is impossible to know whether a goal has been reached. Other criticisms stem from the negative findings of evaluative studies that were designed to measure the impact of casework on such problems as delinquency and gross poverty.[4] In these instances, the optimal goals of reducing delinquency and poverty are unrealistic, not only because the clients who were involved were 'captive' (i.e. they had not asked for a casework service) but also because casework alone, unsupported by other forms of intervention, could not be expected to make more than a modest impact on the lives of clients in such dire circumstances. Other evaluative studies of casework[5] take the view that, to be effective, casework must choose goals that are modest and specific enough to allow worker and client alike to know whether they have been achieved. Those who share this view will be likely to choose goals that other social workers might view as interim or facilitative. For example, one worker might view the reduction of a client's rent arrears as an optimal goal, whereas another with the same client would see it as a goal that is interim to improving the client's role performance as husband and father. The worker with the modest goals might *hope* that the client's success in reducing his rent arrears will help him to achieve the more ambitious goals of the second worker. But the difference between the two workers does not lie in what they *hope* the client will ultimately achieve in life. It lies in their differing views about the appropriate cut-off point for the casework process and their assessment of the capacities of the client. The first worker is likely to have more confidence than the second in the notion that success in one area of a client's life may have a benign effect on others; he may believe that a demonstration of confidence in the client's ability to tackle other problems on his own is more likely to enhance his problem-solving capacities than continuing casework help.

Agency Function
For some social workers, the rationale of their agency demands almost inevitably that goals be stated optimally in terms of personal behaviour. For example, caseworkers in the probation service will want to ensure that their clients do not continue to break the law; caseworkers in local authority social services will want to ensure that clients relate to their children in ways that promote their mental and physical health. However, caseworkers must distinguish between goals that are optimal for agency and client, and goals that are optimal for the casework process. Reid and Epstein point out that many clients for whom an agency has a long-term responsibility require casework help episodically. Examples of this are seen frequently during the crises experienced by people in the initial phases of becoming agency clients when short-term problems must be dealt with, such as obtaining accommodation, getting a job and having debts cleared and children cared for. Subsequently, casework may be vital at other critical points in clients' lives: for children these critical points include entering school, being placed with foster parents and starting work; for adults, they may be crises in personal relationships, serious illnesses and accidents, and problems at work and with official bodies. Activities that the agency and the caseworker engage in outside these critical periods of casework activity should not, in Reid and Epstein's view, be called casework.[6] Such activities may be supervisory, or exercise of the social control functions of the agency; they may be in the nature of routine visits to re-assess the need for further help. Here,

Reid and Epstein define the ingredients that must be present if work with clients is to be considered casework and not something else; the ingredients are the active participation of the client in the casework process and his concurrence with the worker on the goals to be achieved. We shall develop these assumptions later on.

Problems of Clients
It would be reassuring to know that the goals pursued in casework stem logically from an accurate perception of client need. But, in fact, we know that there is not a direct connection between the two. How client need is perceived and defined is in itself a complex subject.[7] Many personal factors influence the client's and worker's perceptions of needs and the ways the worker responds to the need. Other external factors include the already mentioned function of the agency, its resources, policies, and the way its work is organised; and also the policies of other agencies and resources in the wider community. However, it is possible to consider the question of what kinds of needs are susceptible to casework in general, quite apart from these variations in agencies.

Broadly, the problems dealt with by casework can be distinguished in the following four ways:

(1) *Relatively circumscribed problems* affecting delimited areas of a client's life such as obtaining welfare benefits, improving a marital relationship, rehabilitation after a disabling illness and keeping out of trouble with the police. While the effects of the problem may pervade other areas of life, there are not so many other relatively gross problems such as environmental impoverishment and alienation as to militate against the amelioration of the one problem, or to prevent the amelioration from having a benign effect on other problems.

(2) *Relatively severe and pervasive intrapersonal and interpersonal problems* such as alcoholism, gross emotional deprivation and gross lack of social skills. Clients with these problems cannot be helped by the same degree of partialisation of problems as can clients whose problems are more circumscribed. Furthermore, these severe and pervasive problems are often, but not necessarily, linked to equally severe and damaging material deprivation. If the goal is to help them to independence, these clients need a service that is more comprehensive than help with one or two specific problems.

(3) *Relatively long-term problems* requiring continuing concrete services such as care for children and adults, domestic help, and transport to clubs and day centres for handicapped and elderly people.

(4) *Problems resulting from gross material environmental deprivations* shared by many people in a community who are unable to benefit

from any form of help that is not directed first and foremost to improving material conditions in that locality.

These four distinctions are a crude attempt to depict the nature of needs. They are not categorisations of people, nor a typology of target problems.[8] Clients whose problems fall roughly into the first category are excluded from the second and fourth. But otherwise the categories are not mutually exclusive. For example, most parents caring for a handicapped child might be considered to have a relatively circumscribed problem as far as *their* needs are concerned. Yet the problem is also a long-term one that usually requires concrete services as well as personal emotional support. Nor are the distinctions related to categories of clinical diagnosis.[9] However crude, the distinctions are important because they make it possible to relate client need to questions about the appropriateness of casework help, and its general nature and goals.

Let us consider first the issue of appropriateness. Casework is an 'individual remedy'. It must not attempt to pursue goals for which other remedies are better suited. It is certainly inappropriate to deal with problems of the fourth type which require social reform. It is inappropriate also as a means of dealing with problems that are more effectively dealt with at the group, community or organisational levels.[10] With these limitations, we can now consider what kinds of problems social caseworkers can deal with in each of these categories and the kinds of relationships that are required to be developed between workers and clients in order to achieve these different objectives.

(1) In dealing with *relatively circumscribed problems* caseworkers can enhance clients' capabilities to tackle other problems in their lives. The relationship that is required to be developed between caseworker and client is based upon realistic, specific and mutually agreed-upon goals and methods.

(2) By contrast, dealing with *relatively severe intrapersonal and interpersonal problems* makes quite different demands on the caseworker. Because clients suffer from severe and pervasive personal problems which are often combined with gross material deprivation, the caseworker has to consider how these personal problems can be resolved, ameliorated or contained, in addition to making efforts to improve his client's material condition.

Sometimes the intrapersonal problems are dealt with by a psychiatrist or a psycho-therapist. The social worker's task then becomes that of helping the client with interpersonal relationships and to attain material supports. This is typical in the work of social workers located with psychiatric services caring for patients suffering, for example, from chronic neurosis, brain damage, alcoholism and drug addiction. But often it is the *caseworker* and not a psychiatrist who has the major responsibility for influencing the client's intrapersonal life. This is most likely to be true in work with clients who do not manifest symptoms that are susceptible to short-term psychiatric treatment but who nevertheless suffer the effects of gross emotional deprivation. The problem then to be solved is how to provide for the client a nurturing relationship within which he can grow emotionally.

Here, instead of providing a relationship to help the client solve a *particular* problem, the worker must develop a therapeutic relationship through which the client's capacities can be developed on a broad rather than a specific front. It is this particular type of worker–client relationship, in which the client is enabled to experience personal growth, that is most criticised in attacks on casework.

The criticism of therapeutically-oriented casework takes several forms. First, there is the view that caseworkers should not try to provide these relationships themselves but, rather, act as links between clients and significant others who are able to provide authentic relationships. In the case of children it is obvious that parents, foster parents, residential staff, teachers and youth workers fall into this category. It is not so clear as to whom the links can be made in work with adults. But holding this view a caseworker is more likely to encourage an adult to be helped through social group work, and to use family therapy rather than forming the therapeutic relationship himself with the client. For many clients, these would be the treatments of choice. However, some clients who need large amounts of individual attention before being able to benefit from a group may founder on the caseworker's reluctance to be a therapist. In addition, there are some clients who, because of their emotional deprivations, are very destructive in their personal relationships and need a worker who is sufficiently skilled and psychologically indestructible to stay the course.[11]

A second basis for criticism of therapeutic casework is that some caseworkers who attempt to provide nurturing relationships fail to give them sufficient attention. Here, the reservations turn on the question of agency resources and functions, the worker's emotional and technical capacity, and whether his personal characteristics allow him to play a therapeutic role.

Regarding agency resources, a relationship that purports to be therapeutic to which the caseworker gives too little time and attention may be more damaging than none at all. In such a case it is surely more helpful to the client if the relationship is addressed to practical and material difficulties rather than to the more ambitious goal of psychological maturation.

The third kind of criticism that is made of clinical casework relates to the tendency of some caseworkers to make psychological growth the goal of *all* of their work, irrespective of the needs and desires of particular clients. Insofar as this criticism is justified, the fault stems from a failure to make proper distinctions between different client needs. Insights into people's needs that are derived from the residential treatment of disturbed children and from psychoanalysis have, of course, been invaluable to caseworkers, but the goals of these psycho-therapeutic endeavours should not be adopted indiscriminately or unrealistically.

We have dwelt on the needs of clients with severe intrapersonal problems because we think it important not to lose sight of these needs in an era that, rightly, lays stress on the social worker's function in linking clients to material resources and in improving people's problem-solving capacities by way of collective action. There is a danger in the tendency of social-work-in-general and casework-in-particular to swing back and forth between the two extremes of great concern with people's psychological/emotional experience and concern with people's access to material and cultural resources. Rather like two sides of the same coin, casework-as-a-whole must reflect both concerns with equal intensity.[12]

(3) *Relatively long-term problems requiring concrete service*: our third category is concerned with the needs of people who are recipients of services like residential care and daycare, home help, fostering, meals-on-wheels, and aids for the handicapped. These services can be viewed in two ways. First they can be seen as no different from other services such as health services, education, transport and the services of an electrician, plumber and motor mechanic. These are services that people buy or, through taxation, services to which they have a right. To be a recipient of these services does not imply the need of a caseworker. When services are thus institutionalised and become part of society's way of providing for the welfare of all citizens it is possible for people to use them without stigma and to negotiate for them without the help of a caseworker acting as broker or mediator to establish eligibility.

With the alternative view, these services are perceived as residual; that is, they are considered to be services specifically for people who, for varying reasons, fail to make adequate use of society's normal provision. With this view the need for casework is considered to be the rule rather than the exception.

In reality most services are based on a mixture of institutional and residual conceptions of need, and agencies differ considerably in their propensity to allocate a caseworker to every applicant. When an agency is not offering a comprehensive service the place of casework is easier to determine. For example, services run by the erstwhile children's departments were for the most part clearly residual, whereas health and welfare departments in local authorities had the makings of a non-residual service.

It is our contention that if a social service is delivered in a manner that meets individual need and enhances the recipient's self-esteem, there is no role for a caseworker unless:

(a) The applicant's problem is obscure and there is need for a skilled assessment to determine what kind of a service is appropriate.
(b) While receiving the service the client needs casework help to solve related social/emotional/economic problems. In the context of a long period of service there may be several 'episodes' of casework help.
(c) The client's need is for the kind of 'nurturing' relationship we have discussed above and the service being received such as aids for a handicapped person or a child-minding service does not include it.

Unfortunately, services are not always delivered in a manner that meets individual need and enhances self-esteem, and in these instances there is an important role for the caseworker as mediator or advocate; or, alternatively, as enabler to the client in helping him to negotiate for the kind of service he wants.[13]

Cormack and McDougall[14] make a useful distinction between casework proper and the use of casework principles in social service agencies. By casework principles they were referring to the following beliefs: that the individual is an end in himself; that the giving of a service should be a process of social co-operation; that the service must be designed to enhance independence; and that workers must be scrupulous about the way in which they obtain and use knowledge of the individual applicant's life, circumstances and problems. They argue strongly for the embodiment of these principles in the structure of all social services, including income maintenance, health and housing. They indicate that the use of casework proper is for people who have needs that extend *beyond* what the general service is designed to meet. With the expansion of service provision in what might be thought of as the social work sector of local authorities this distinction is important to maintain.

(4) *The need for environmental improvement in a neighbourhood*: insofar as our final category of problems – *gross material environmental deprivations* – is related to casework, it brings us to the question of the integration of casework and community work. Casework as a method on its own cannot make an impact on problems arising from slum conditions, lack of play space, poor delivery of public services and bad maintenance of housing. As we have noted, people suffering from such deprivations need a response other than the 'individual remedy'. Economic and social factors rather than psychological factors may be depriving them of adequate material and educational resources. Hartman points out that when adequate services are available, but for some reason are not accessible to particular clients, casework methods include individual-

ising and co-ordinating the services and enabling the client to use them; but when services are not available, are being withheld or are delivered in a dehumanising way, caseworkers may get into the business of developing services, mediating, advocating and participating with clients to bring about small-scale social change.[15] In our view, methods such as mediation and advocacy are proper to casework when it is appropriate to effect an 'individual remedy'. But when such activities are performed on behalf of groups of clients, or when caseworkers engage in resource development and small-scale community development, they are not engaged in social casework. It may be group work or community work.

In practice, of course, the boundaries between one modality and another can become blurred when the same worker in the course of a day moves from work with a family needing help with their supplementary benefits, to work with a group of clients aiming to start a claimants' union, to work with a housing association aiming to increase accommodation for handicapped people. The fact that the worker might *think* of himself primarily as a caseworker does not mean that all of his *activities* are casework. Only his work that day with the family can properly be called casework.

Goldberg's[16] micro-level intervention model emphasising the social worker's role in meeting human needs through structural rather than individual change depicts a practitioner who is able to range over work with individuals and families, work with groups of clients on behalf of themselves and others, and work with others on behalf of clients. She emphasises the importance of looking beyond each client to see if there are others facing the same task, and of the worker acting on the logic of what he sees. In effect, she depicts a generalist worker using a unitary method of practice and she does not use the words 'casework', 'group work' and 'community work' to describe any part of the worker's total activity.

Goldberg begs the kind of educational and organisational questions we discuss in Chapters 13 and 14, but nevertheless succeeds in clarifying greatly the point at which 'the individual remedy' is inappropriate with respect to the needs of groups of people suffering material deprivations. Insofar as there may be individuals and families within those groups needing individualised personal help, it should be given concurrently with intervention at group, organisational and community levels.

FACTORS INFLUENCING THE PROFESSIONAL'S MODE OF PRACTICE

Critiques of social casework often give the impression that there exists a theoretically orthodox version of practice. But the truth is exactly the opposite. There is a variety of theoretical and pragmatic approaches to casework, some of which differ in fundamental respects. Examples include the diagnostic and the functional approaches, the psychodynamic and the behaviourist approaches. Moreover, any particular theoretical stance adopted by one segment of casework does not assure that there will be consistency in practice within that segment.

Empirical evidence suggests that the worker's characteristic ways of thinking and relating are a far more potent determinant of his practice methods and techniques than the character, needs and the cultural background of the particular client with whom he works.[17] The worker's values and personal style may account for his preference for a particular theoretical approach.

The division that appears to be the most significant one among practitioners is the great divide between workers who aim at a clear and explicit definition of casework goals to achieve a mutually agreed upon and planned intervention and workers who are concerned with the more existential qualities of their encounters with clients, whether long-term or time-limited; for these workers the experience of the relationship is the crucial element that enables the client to deal with his problems.

These differences may reflect both differences in theory and differences in the personal characteristics of the worker. For example, it is possible to have a psychoanalytical orientation and yet, by differentiating between the ways in which the theory is used in psychoanalysis and in casework, to believe either in the importance of arriving at shared, explicitly-defined goals or in the importance of learning through the manipulation of the worker–client relationship.

There is some evidence that supports the view that casework is most effective when the goals that are pursued by the worker are clear to, and agreed upon by, the client; and when the duration of the casework process is time-limited (i.e. when the number of interviews and/or the date of termination are fixed at the outset).[18] There is also significant evidence that success in casework is determined by three intrinsic characteristics of the worker, namely, the worker's *warmth, ability to empathise* with the client and his *authenticity*. 'Authenticity' in this context refers to the extent to which the sentiments he expresses verbally to the client are congruent with the sentiments he conveys by subtler non-verbal and usually unconscious processes.[19] Carkhuff in 1969 added a fourth characteristic to the list of those considered to be crucial to a helping relationship, namely, that the worker be *action-oriented*.[20] Warmth, empathy and authenticity are the determinants of success that one would expect to have been identified by the open-ended, existential school of thought rather than by those who support a time-limited, goal-oriented, task-centred type of casework. They are the characteristics associated with Carl Rogers's client-centred therapy which emphasises the importance of the worker picking up the verbal clues that the client gives him and going with the client down whatever avenue of thought the clues may lead to. However, these characteristics of the worker can be given equal stress in work that is time-limited and goal-oriented. The worker may have to make difficult judgements about how far he should travel with the client down avenues that look like diversions from the main goal. But the difficulty is one of degree because it is certainly present to some extent in a client-centred approach.

In our view, warmth, empathy and authenticity are crucial ingredients in any helping relationship and they must be present in any casework that is effective *no matter what the theoretical orientation*. In the training of caseworkers it is certainly right to pay considerable attention to the enhancement of these characteristics in the student, for without them the student is bound to fail. And as we have noted above, for many clients the relationship with a caseworker is not *per se* the main instrument of change, but a means of engaging in collaborative problem-solving. To believe, in addition, that the needs of some clients are best met by work that focuses on specific goals is not to devalue the importance of the worker's personality and his understanding of human relationships. Client-oriented and goal-oriented work do not have attributes that are mutually exclusive. It is useful, rather, to contrast work that reduces ambiguity between worker and client (whether in terms of goals or relationships or both) with work that tends to heighten ambiguity because of lack of communication on the part of the worker as to goals, role expectations and his assessment of the availability of resources to effect the change that the client wishes.[21]

Apart from the difference between workers who believe that it is important to specify goals early on in the casework process and those who do not, workers differ in their preferences for different types of goals. This preference is, to some extent, associated with the congruity of the worker's personal values and style with particular theoretical orientations. For some workers the influence of a particular theoretical orientation is manifestly strong. Others are not so tightly reined by a particular theory and, in effect, are more eclectic.[22] Let us turn now to a consideration of some of these theories.

Theories that Influence Practice
It is not possible to discuss all of the theories that have influenced social casework practice. However, since so much criticism of casework has centred on a supposed exclusive reliance on psychoanalytic theory it is important to begin by discussing the place of psychoanalytic theory in British casework.

The extent to which psychoanalytic theory has been a major influence in casework has certainly been exaggerated. Even in the United States,

Alexander[23] has challenged the historical accuracy of the view that in the 1920s the influence of Freudian theory was responsible for an undue emphasis on personality change. His careful review of the social work literature of that decade supports the notion that Freudian theory was familiar only to an elite few and that the more sociological approach of Mary Richmond[24] informed the bulk of social work practice.

In this country psychoanalytic theory was introduced into the education of social workers after 1929 with the beginning of the mental health course at the London School of Economics. The number of workers qualifying from this course as psychiatric social workers was initially small and, although they were later to become influential, they were not purveyors of an exclusively psychoanalytical orientation. Following on their education in social administration, the mental health course taught students psychology and psychological medicine from a wide and often conflicting range of theory.

In actual practice, the kind of theory on which the students subsequently drew was determined more by the kind of agency in which they worked than anything else. Child guidance was a field of practice that relied almost exclusively on psychoanalytic and analytic theory.[25] Child psychiatrists undoubtedly influenced British social work but they probably made less impact outside the worlds of child guidance and child care than within them.

Social workers who identified strongly with the psychoanalytic movement may well have approximated their style more closely to that of the psychoanalyst than to that of the problem-solving counsellor.[26] It is important to distinguish between social workers who based some of their *knowledge* of human growth and behaviour on psychoanalytic theory and those who actually *used* a psychoanalytic approach on their own or in association with psychoanalysts.

These latter, in relating to clients, tended to play a passive role, to make explicit use of the transference and, where appropriate, to aim to develop the client's insight into hitherto unconscious processes. It is this style of casework which is currently under fire. But often the critical onslaught fails to discriminate sufficiently between the treatment method of the psychoanalyst which, in its entirety, has been considered inappropriate by most social workers, and *the use of psychoanalytic theory in enhancing the social worker's understanding of clients and of themselves*, and in guiding decisions about action to be taken during the casework process.[27]

Apart from psychoanalytic theory, casework draws now on a wide range of theories stemming from experimental psychology and from various types of psycho-social therapy practised with individuals and groups. It also draws on social systems theory, communications theory, role theory and other sociological theories.[28] Among the many psychotherapies that have influenced casework, two in particular should be singled out as having a special influence on British casework: behaviour modification and family therapy.

The behavioural learning theory approach to casework has recently come to the fore as the result of evaluative studies comparing the results of psychoanalytically-oriented psychotherapy with those of behaviour therapy in the treatment of specific disorders and problem behaviour.[29] Transposed to casework these studies suggest that the behavioural approach may be exceedingly effective in the resolution of specific behavioural difficulties that appear to be otherwise intractable such as phobias, enuresis, psycho-sexual difficulties and certain forms of aggressive behaviour. Practitioners of behaviour modification will therefore make the resolution of these difficulties the focus of their work and the 'optimal' goal for the treatment process.

Critics of the approach tend to complain of its too-narrow focus and limited goals; that it only deals with the 'symptoms' of underlying problems. They fear its potential for being used unethically. The last complaint, however, applies to all forms of treatment, the only caveat being that the more effective the treatment the greater the risk entailed in its unethical use. The narrowness of focus and the limits of its goals may well account for its effectiveness. The fact that there is a relationship between degree of specificity of goals and degree of success of treatment supports what was said earlier about the need in casework for realistic goals upon which the client can agree.

Apart from the clinical use of learning theory, caseworkers may use it in ways that are analogous to the non-clinical use of psychoanalytic theory; that is, it may be used to enhance understanding of human behaviour and to guide action in the casework process. In this respect, learning theory represents the 'commonsense' approach to influencing behaviour. It need not rely on reinforcement schedules or de-sensitisation techniques but on responses such as personal encouragement of appropriate behaviour and the withdrawal of personal attention from inappropriate behaviour; and also on a variety of techniques such as modelling and behavioural rehearsal which are often used by caseworkers who may be unaware of their roots in learning theory but perform them intuitively.[30]

Family therapy, which is increasingly capturing the interest of caseworkers, has its theoretical roots in anthropological and sociological studies of the family as well as in psychoanalytic theory, small group theory, general systems theory, kinetics and communications theory. It is in a sense a hybrid of family casework and group therapy. Clearly the caseworker treating the family-as-a-whole needs to have group work skills in addition to substantial knowledge of family relationships. As with other recent developments in individual work, there is a phenomenological emphasis in family therapy, a tendency to focus on the interaction taking place in the therapeutic session rather than on events in the past or events occurring outside the session. Therapy is usually terminated when a change in communication patterns and role relations has taken place.[31]

The family therapist's view of the family as an interacting system tends to make this the treatment of choice in all cases where individual problems are generated and supported by other family members as well as by an individual client's own inner drives. Because the difficulties of so many social work clients are of this nature, social workers are increasingly expressing the belief that more family treatment should be available, and many professionals are seeking training in family therapy.

The goal of family therapy is to change role relations in the family in such a way as to free individual members from having to engage in pathologically induced and supported role behaviour. Most frequently it is the children who are freed by modifications occurring in the parents' marital relationship and by modifications in parent–child relationships.[32]

The final theoretical orientation that we shall mention is social systems theory. It has been discussed earlier in 'Divisions and unifications in social work practice' (Chapter 3). Although it has not been greatly referred to in relation to casework until recent years, Lutz used it as a major theoretical framework in his conceptualisation of casework in 1956.[33] This theoretical approach does not offer a guide to specific strategies and techniques but, rather, it provides a conceptual framework that helps the caseworker to decide where intervention should most appropriately occur: for example, should intervention focus on the individual, the family, external systems (e.g. employers, schools and medical services) or at the point of interaction between the client system and the external system? The caseworker with a social systems orientation is more likely than other practitioners to intervene with external systems in an attempt to strengthen the client's environmental resources. But in addition to this indirect form of helping, the social systems orientation is also crucial to direct helping in family systems.

DISTINGUISHING FEATURES OF CASEWORK

In the introduction to this chapter we said that opinion has varied as to what constitutes the core of casework. In discussing the varied goals of casework and the different theoretical orientations upon which it draws, we have tried to show that casework cannot be identified by a particular set of goals or a particular theoretical orientation. However, we do believe that there are characteristics of casework that distinguish it from other forms of work with individuals and families.[34]

Decision Making as to Goals and Methods

An important feature of casework practice is the caseworker's concern to involve the client in setting goals and planning the means for problem solving. However, there are many people whom caseworkers might wish to help who do not wish to change their lives; and there are others who might wish for change, but not by involving themselves with a caseworker. Some caseworkers therefore spend a large amount of time reaching out to people who are potential but not actual clients. Vagrants, addicts, delinquents and poor and disorganised families are examples of client groups who typically need time to gain trust in the caseworker before they can agree about the need for change and its goals. Strictly speaking, the potential client should not be considered an actual client until he has decided to work with the caseworker towards particular ends. Only in these circumstances can joint decision making occur.

Sometimes the caseworker will fail to achieve a working contract with a potential client. But successful or not, the attempt to develop a relationship in which the client will participate in deciding how to improve his life is all part of casework. By contrast, casework is not being done when professionals do not consider joint decision making as a central focus. Examples of work have already been mentioned that, however valuable, are not casework. These include the delivery of a service which has already been agreed upon by the agency and the client such as transport to a club, care in an old people's home, child minding; maintaining contact with individuals such as registered handicapped people for whom the agency has some statutory responsibility; exercising social control functions of the agency outside the context of a significant relationship, such as may happen in statutory work with delinquents and the mentally ill. It is often stated that the use of authority does not nullify a casework relationship. Rather, it is a crucial part of it. But it should be emphasised that however fragile the casework relationship, casework nonetheless presumes client participation. The mere presence of a qualified caseworker on the scene does not automatically transform the exercise of external constraints into 'casework'.

Sometimes the personal delivery of a practical service by the social worker is another equally crucial part of a casework process. Often, the practical help is given by a worker other than the caseworker who decided with the client what service was needed. While this may contribute to the helping process, the non-caseworker, however skilled, is not doing casework.

Sometimes, social workers carry out procedures that have been administratively determined. But, although professional judgement may be exercised in carrying out these procedures, if neither the worker nor the client has any part to play in deciding whether the procedure is appropriate to the case, this is not casework. Illustrations of this are workers complying with agency regulations to visit certain categories of vulnerable people at specified intervals, and checking up to see that requirements laid down by statute are observed, such as the boarding-out regulations for children in care. Britton quotes a more evocative and now defunct example from the Poor Law Act 1930, which laid down that the local authority should set to work and put out as apprentices all children whose parents could not maintain them. She contrasts this with the wording of the Children Act 1948 which states that each child is to be helped in such a way as to 'further his best interests'.[35] If social work with individuals and families is to be casework, then there must be options as to ends and means left open to both worker and client.

The Use of Relationship
The joint decision making process is an essential part of casework and it is one of the necessary features of what has come to be honoured as the 'relationship between client and worker'. The integrity of joint decision making depends on each party's capacity for an authentic exchange of viewpoints. Outside a reasonably sound relationship this requirement is difficult for most people to realise. Here we return to the importance of the relationship as a prerequisite to successful problem solving.

The other aspect of the casework relationship that we have mentioned is its use as a therapeutic tool. We have already touched on the hazards and issues involved. But undoubtedly, for a large number of clients, the development of a growth-inducing relationship is crucial to their progress. Here, one must distinguish between the warmth and concern that most social workers bring to all of their relationships, and the conscious drawing on knowledge of human behaviour and its meaning in particular circumstances in order to adapt one's behaviour in specific and subtle detail to meet a specific client's needs. The warmth and concern of the first kind is crucial to any form of help whether in establishing eligibility for a service, providing practical help or comforting the bereaved. Of itself, it does not constitute casework. By contrast, the conscious use of a relationship is a skill that validates those who have it as caseworkers. Without it a worker may be able to individualise the service as far as the client's outer needs are concerned but cannot individualise his own behaviour to meet his client's inner needs.[36]

Casework Compared with Social Group Work and Community Work
Much that has been said about joint decision making and the importance of the relationship with the client system is analogous to practice in modalities other than casework. However, as the client system becomes larger and the work more indirect (i.e. as we move into the realm of broad service provision and social planning), the importance of understanding and providing for specific individuals decreases. It is this

emphasis which accounts for the caseworker's concentration on inter-personal behaviour, mental states and the psychological effects of social misfortune. Skill in human relations is, of course, crucial to community workers as well as to caseworkers, but the *detailed* knowledge of inter-personal dynamics that is essential to the caseworker is of little practical value to the community worker dealing with common problems. This is not to suggest that the community worker can do without knowledge of individual psychology, nor that the caseworker can do without socio-logical knowledge and knowledge of political science. But the *degree* of knowledge required in each practice modality must depend on how it is applied.

One other difference between caseworkers and other social work prac-titioners relates to the nature of the caseworker's interaction with an individual as opposed to a group. In a group, the person who looks after the expressive needs and the person who keeps the focus of attention on the task need not be one and the same. The group worker can assume either role. In casework with an individual, the caseworker must carry both roles, and these often conflict.[37] This conflict is especially felt in the practice of task-centred casework, but in varying degrees is present in all forms of individual helping. This is one of the reasons for the emphasis given in developing caseworkers' skills in forming relationships that are required to withstand the most unpropitious circumstances.

In summary of all the intricate facets of casework that we have per-force lightly touched on, we end by quoting from a work offering severe and pungent criticisms of the way in which casework is often practised. Briar and Miller write in their Introduction:

'Social casework is a unique enterprise. No other profession has taken the individual person so seriously, nor has made the promotion of each person's particular aspirations and potentialities its primary function, nor has set as its cardinal principle the notion that each person deserves respect and dignity, no matter how offensive he may seem. Other professions and enterprises share some or all of these commitments, but none have made of them their central purpose. These are lofty and therefore fragile and elusive objectives. So per-haps casework can be forgiven for the conspicuous discrepancies between goals and performance that sometimes appear in practice.[38]

NOTES AND REFERENCES FOR CHAPTER 7

1 See, for example: E. M. Goldberg *et al.*, *Helping the Aged* (London: George Allen & Unwin, 1970); William J. Reid and Ann W. Shyne, *Brief and Ex-tended Casework* (New York: Columbia University Press, 1969).

2 See, for example: R. W. Roberts and R. H. Nee (eds), *Theories of Social Casework* (Chicago: University of Chicago Press, 1970); Richmond, *What Is*

Social Casework?; Cherry Morris (ed.), *Social Casework in Great Britain* (London: Faber, 1950); Swithun Bowers, 'The nature and definition of casework', in *Principles and Techniques in Social Casework* (New York: Family Service Association of America, 1950); Gordon Hamilton, *Theory and Practice of Social Casework* (New York: Columbia University Press, 1952); Virginia P. Robinson, *A Changing Psychology in Social Casework* (Chapel Hill: University of North Carolina Press, 1930); W. J. Reid and Laura Epstein, *Task Centred Casework* (New York: Columbia University Press, 1972).

3 Goldstein, *Social Work Practice*, pp. 160–2.

4 See, for example: E. J. Mullen, R. M. Chazin and D. M. Feldstein, *Preventing Chronic Dependency* (New York: Community Service Society of New York, 1970); D. Wallace, 'The Chemung County evaluation of casework service to dependent multi-problem families', *Social Service Review*, vol. XLI, no. 4 (1967).

5 See, for example, Goldberg *et al.*, *Helping the Aged*; Reid and Epstein, *Task Centred Casework*.

6 Reid and Epstein, *Task Centred Casework*, pp. 201–15.

7 See, for example: Gilbert Smith and Robert Harris, 'Ideologies of need and the organisation of social work departments', *British Journal of Social Work*, vol. II, no. 1 (Spring, 1972); Jonathan Bradshaw, 'The concept of social need', *New Society* (30 March 1972).

8 For an example of a typology of target problems, see Reid and Epstein, *Task Centred Casework*, ch. 3.

9 See Jean Nursten, *Process of Casework* (London: Pitman, 1974), for an account of casework based on the matching of type of intervention to diagnostic categories in psychological medicine.

10 See, for example: Una Cormack and Kay McDougall, 'Casework in social service', in Morris (ed.), *Social Casework in Great Britain*, pp. 20–1; Goldberg *et al.*, *Helping the Aged*, pp. 193–5.

11 Elizabeth E. Irvine, 'The function and use of relationship between client and worker', *British Journal of Psychiatric Social Work*, vol. II, no. 6 (June 1952).

12 See, for example: A. M. Laquer, 'The caseworker's task in meeting the client's inner and outer needs', *British Journal of Psychiatric Social Work*, no. 10 (1954); Edgar Myers, 'The caseworker's problems in meeting the inner and outer needs of clients', *British Journal of Psychiatric Social Work*, no. 10 (1954).

13 Goldberg *et al.*, *Helping the Aged*, pp. 114–21.

14 Cormack and McDougall, 'Casework in social service', pp. 31–5.

15 Hartman, 'But what is social casework?', pp. 411–19.

16 Gale Goldberg, 'Structural approach to practice: a new model', *Social Work* (New York: March 1974), pp. 150–5.

17 W. J. Reid, 'Characteristics of casework intervention', *Welfare in Review*, no. 8 (1967) and 'A study of caseworkers' use of insight-oriented techniques', *Social Casework*, no. 1 (1967); J. Schmidt, 'The use of purpose in casework', *Social Work*, no. 1 (1969). (The studies are referred to by Goldstein in *Social Work Practice*, pp. 57–8.)

18 See, for example: Reid and Shyne, *Brief and Extended Casework*; J. M. Rosenfeld, 'Strangeness between helper and client: a possible explanation of non-use of professional help', *Social Service Review* (March 1964).

19 C. B. Truax and R. R. Carkhuff, *Toward Effective Counselling and Psychotherapy* (Chicago: Aldine, 1967).

20 For a discussion of this, see Margaret Yelloly, 'The helping relationship', in Derek Jehu *et al.*, *Behaviour Modification in Social Work* (New York: Wiley, 1972), ch. 6, pp. 152–60.

21 John E. Mayer and Noel Timms, *The Client Speaks* (London: Routledge & Kegan Paul, 1970), pp. 138–48.

22 See, for example, Barbara Hudson, 'An inadequate personality', *Social Work Today*, vol. VI, no. 16, pp. 506–8.

23 Leslie B. Alexander, 'Social work's Freudian deluge: myth or reality?', *Social Service Review* (December 1972).

24 Mary Richmond, *Social Diagnosis* (New York: Russell Sage Foundation, 1917).

25 There were also, of course, always a number of influential Jungians as well as Freudians in this field.

26 See, for example, Margaret L. Ferard and Noel K. Hunnybun, *The Case-worker's Use of Relationships* (London: Tavistock Publications, 1962), pp. 48–81.

27 For a discussion of these issues, see: Elizabeth E. Irvine, 'Transference and reality in the casework relationship', *British Journal of Psychiatric Social Work*, vol. III, no. 4 (1956); Margaret Yelloly, 'The concept of insight', in Derek Jehu *et al.*, *Behaviour Modification in Social Work*, ch. 5, pp. 126–49.

28 Recent summaries include: Raymond Corsini (ed.), *Current Psychotherapies* (Itasca, Ill.: Peacock, 1973); James Whittaker, *Social Treatment*, ch. 4, pp. 62–109 and Appendix, pp. 200–47; R. W. Roberts and R. H. Nee (eds), *Theories of Social Casework*.

29 See, for example: V. Meyer and Edward Chesser, *Behaviour Therapy in Clinical Psychiatry* (London: Penguin, 1970); R. P. Hawkins *et al.*, 'Behaviour therapy in the home: amelioration of problem parent–child relations with the parent in a therapeutic role', *Journal of Experimental Psychology*, no. 4, pp. 99–107.

30 For full accounts of behaviour modification in social work, see: Derek Jehu, *Learning Theory and Social Work* (London: Routledge & Kegan Paul, 1967); Derek Jehu *et al.*, *Behaviour Modification in Social Work*; Edwin Thomas, *The Socio-Behavioural Approach and Applications to Social Work* (New York: Council on Social Work Education, 1967).

31 Donald Bloch and Kitty LaPerriere, *Techniques in Family Psychotherapy: A Primer* (New York: Grune & Stratton, 1973), ch. 1.

32 For a study of family therapy, see the works of N. W. Ackerman, S. Minuchin and V. Satir; also: A. C. R. Skynner, 'A group-analytic approach to conjoint family therapy', *Social Work Today*, vol. II, no. 8 (15 July 1971); 'Indications for and against conjoint family therapy', *Social Work Today*, vol. II, no. 7 (1 July 1971).

33 Werner A. Lutz, *Concepts and Principles Underlying Social Casework Practice* (New York: National Association of Social Workers, May 1956).

34 Ron Baker, 'The challenge of British casework', *Social Work Today*, vol. IV, no. 10 (7 August 1973).

35 Clare Britton, 'Child Care', in Morris (ed.), *Social Casework in Great Britain*, p. 170.

36 See, for example: E. M. Goldberg, 'The function and use of relationship in psychiatric social work', *British Journal of Psychiatric Social Work*, no. 8 (November 1953); Irvine, 'The function and use of relationship between client and psychiatric social worker'.

37 Mary E. Burns and Paul H. Glasser, 'Similarities and differences in casework and group work practice', *Social Service Review*, vol. XXXVII, no. 4 (December 1963).

38 Scott Briar and Henry Miller, *Problems and Issues in Social Casework* (New York: Columbia University Press, 1971), pp. v–vi.

Chapter 8

SOCIAL GROUP WORK MODELS: POSSESSION AND HERITAGE*

Beulah Rothman and Catherine P. Papell

The social group work method, like all social work methods, has developed largely experientially. Yet it has done so within a framework of some kind of guiding consensus about its essential elements. Persistently, social group workers have sought to formulate a logical relationship between these elements and pragmatic solutions to the tasks that have confronted them in practice. The evolutionary efforts of group workers to describe repeated patterns of phenomena and to define practice, in the language of science, has resulted in the emergence of several different theoretical models of social group work method. We have arrived at that stage of theory construction that can now be identified as model building.

A theoretical model is described by Kogan as 'a scheme or map for "making sense" out of the portion of the real world' in relation to which the worker is seeking to act.[1] A model is a conceptual design to solve a problem that exists in reality. A model orders those elements in a given universe that are relevant to solve the problem. Higher levels of generalisation or theory can be formulated when relationships hypothesised from a model are found to apply to a multitude of problems involving similar elements.

In our opinion, three models for social group work method can now be identified. The sequence of emergence of these models is elusive. Rudiments of these models are found scattered historically throughout the development of group work. Each has had periods of ascendant or waning commitment as practitioners have responded to the social scene and innovative calls for our professional services.

A core problem to which each model is addressed is concerned in some way with the central search of all social work to identify its societal functions. One model tells us that our first priority is provision and prevention. A second model prefers restoration and rehabilitation. A

* Reprinted with permission of the authors from *Education for Social Work*, no. 2 (Autumn 1966).

third model attempts to encompass and reconcile these two historical streams. Thus our present state of theory building is but one of the several efforts within the broader arena of the professional struggle to establish a relationship between our methods and our service to society.

The question of function is intertwined with a second problem of major import. Historically in group work theory and in its practice there has existed the eternal triangle of the individual, the small group and the larger society. These three have presented themselves as significant ingredients to be considered in any theoretical formulation, but the appropriate balance of each to the others has never been resolved. Thus, when one theoretical formulation tends to stress the individual, professional criticism is raised loudly from many quarters. When a formulation emerges that gives precedence to either of the other two factors, a similar reaction can be observed. The writers are not free of bias in regard to this triad. In our conjecture of the models that have emerged, a review of each will call attention to the gap or emphasis given these three integral parts.

It is perhaps the determination to resolve these two central problems, function and focus, that has deterred the development of a unified model for social group work, but has at the same time reaffirmed the common threads of our history. The three models that we describe and examine in this paper we shall henceforth identify by the following designations:

> (1) The social goals model.
> (2) The remedial model.
> (3) The reciprocal model.

In order to grasp the attributes and characteristics distinguishing these three models, we shall address ourselves to the following three levels of inquiry:[2]

(1) How does the model define the function of social group work?
  Who is the client to be served by the method?
  How does the model view the group as the unit of service?
  What is the image of the professional role?
  What is the nature of the agency auspice through which the group work service is rendered?
(2) What are the knowledge sources that serve as theoretical foundations for the model?
(3) What practice principles are generated by the model? Since it is necessary to limit the scope of this chapter, we shall be concerned primarily with practice principles that pertain to assessment and implementation.

THE SOCIAL GOALS MODEL

Before proceeding with discussions of the social goals model, it must be understood that this model does not exist as a single formulation in our literature. It is not identified with a central theoretician who has systematically set forth all its elements. It is, in fact, a model that has its origins in the earliest traditions of professional group work practice. The central problems with which the social goals model attempts to deal are those related to the social order and the social value orientation in small groups. Historically, youth-serving organisations, settlements and Jewish community centres relied heavily on this model in developing and promoting group work services.

The early writings of such foremost thinkers as Coyle, Kaiser, Phillips, Konopka, Cohen, Miller, Ginsberg, Wilson and Klein provide essential concepts and connecting propositions which, when combined, can be said to have produced this model. None of these writers would subscribe to this model in its entirety. In fact, several are clearly identified with the other two. However, each could find in the social goals model some piece that could be identified as his contribution and commitment.

The social goals model, although emerging from our past, has not been discarded. Interestingly, the model has been reaffirmed as critical strains have developed in the larger society. During the war era, the McCarthy era, and now during the period of struggle for integration, world peace and economic opportunity, this model has been presenting itself for use. Rooted as it is in the value system of our profession, every new effort at theoretical formulation of group work method either incorporates something of this model or is subjected to criticism in relation to it. Since 1962 a striking revival of interest in this model is evident. The University of Pittsburgh's recent position paper challenges the strains in the profession that seem to be abandoning this model.[3] Hyman J. Wiener's work has produced a new level of theoretical sophistication in restatement of the model.[4]

Key concepts in the social goals model are 'social consciousness' and 'social responsibility'. The function of social group work is to create a broader base of knowledgeable and skilled citizenry. 'It is our role and function,' state Ginsberg and Goldberg, to bring about 'discussions of social issues . . . to help define action alternatives which in turn, hopefully result in informed political and social action'.[5]

The model assumes that there is a unity between social action and individual psychological health. Every individual is seen as potentially capable of some form of meaningful participation in the mainstream of society. Thus the social goals model regards the individual as being in need of opportunity and assistance in revitalising his drive towards others in a common cause and in converting self-seeking into social contribution. The therapeutic implications of social participation make the application of this model available to group work practice with groups of varying illness and health. In describing a social action project at Camarillo State Hospital, Joseph D. Jacobs illustrates the use of the social goals model in a treatment setting.[6]

Consistent with its view of the individual, the social goals model approaches every group as possessing a potential for affecting social change. Programme development moves toward uncovering this strength in the group, with social action as the desired outcome. This potential derives from the assumption that collective group action represents individual social competence.

The social goals model views the worker as an 'influence'[7] person with responsibility, according to Wiener, for 'the cultivation of social consciousness in groups . . . elevated to the same priority as . . . developing closer interpersonal relations'.[8] Wiener speaks of this as the 'political man approach'.[9] He goes on to say, however, that the group worker 'does not attempt to dictate a particular political view but does seek to inculcate a value system'.[10] The group worker personifies the values of social responsibility and serves as a role model for the client, stimulating and reinforcing modes of conduct appropriate to citizenship responsibility directed toward social change.

The social goals model primarily envisions group work services at a community level and agency as an integral part of the neighbourhood. The setting is accessible and flexible in offering institutional auspices for a variety of collective efforts. It responds to the interests of various segments of the community and is willing to initiate and recruit for social action. The agency then becomes the vehicle through which members may acquire instrumental skills in social action and institutional support for communal change. The social goals model does not set up priorities for services but insists that such priorities develop out of the particular needs of the community at a given moment in time. Grappling with agency policies or agency limitations is not regarded as a deterrent to client strength. Rather it is the fabric from which practitioners and their clients learn to 'test the limits of authority and sanction, demonstrating that sanction is the product of an ongoing process – constantly evolving and often susceptible to more influence than we think'.[11]

Furthermore, the agency conveys the value that increased leisure time shall be harnessed for the common good and not solely for individual enrichment.

Since the social goals model in the past has been reliant more on ideology than on science, its theoretical underpinnings have only recently become more apparent. It would appear that neo-Freudian personality theories have been utilised in attaching importance to cultural differences and to the significance of interpersonal relations. A significant degree of individual and group malfunctioning is attributable to the malfunctioning of the social system. From the newer body of sociological theory the model picks up on opportunity theory and on theories of powerlessness, cultural deprivation and inter-generational alienation. Current treatment theories of crisis and primary prevention are congenial to this model. The theories still to be seen exerting most influence on the model are theories of economic and political democracy and the educational philosophies of Dewey, Kilpatrick and Lindeman, particularly with regard to conceptions of leadership, communal responsibility and forms of group interaction.

To deal with the external environment of the group, the social goals model has generated a large body of principles designed to activate the group in relation to agency and community. Clarification of agency policy, positive use of limitations, identification with agency goals, determination of appropriate issues for collective action and the weighting of alternatives for action and their consequences are all familiar principles heavily relied on in the social goals model. Furthermore, assessment and implementation with regard to the individual do not have to await intensive study of each member. The worker's assessment is first directed toward understanding normative behaviours manifested in the group as representative of the life style of the community and its subcultures. It is against this background that individual assessment can be formulated with respect to self-image, identity, social skill, knowledge of environmental resources and leadership potential. Principles related to the group emphasise participation, consensus and group task.

It is understandable that considerable explication of practice principles is to be found in recent writings pertaining to inter-group relations. We cite the work of Eleanor Ryder[12] and Jack Wiener.[13] In their papers they set forth principles which tell us how and when to make use of supraordinate goals to bring groups together, how to reduce the threat to individuals in heterogeneous groups, and how to engage members in inter-racial activities through a sequence of orderly and manageable steps. On a somewhat different level, but of major importance in this model, are those principles related to self-awareness and professional discipline, particularly with regard to the value system and life style of the worker. It is interesting to note that the transfer of leadership from the professional to the indigenous leadership is implied in this model. Yet specific practice principles dealing with this aspect are noticeably absent in the literature.

A serious shortcoming of the social goals model is that it has not produced a theoretical design that is adequate to meet the problems facing practitioners in all areas of service. Its underemphasis on individual dynamics and its lack of attention to a wide range of individual need leave the practitioner without guidelines for carrying out a social work function with client groups where individual problems take precedence over social problems. It is difficult to see how this model would serve (except by distortion) to provide a basis for social group work practice with 'admission' or 'discharge' groups in a mental hospital.

Each of the models places the social group work method in some relationship to the other social work methods. The social goals model tends to move group work toward community organisation method, but in so doing further obscures the boundaries between them. Ambiguity is particularly evident when group-serving agencies increasingly call upon grass roots membership to solve community problems, sometimes in the name of the group work method and other times in the name of community organisation method.

One last comment must be made about the social goals model. The principles of democratic group process that are fundamental to this model have become the hallmark of all social group work practice. Every practitioner, regardless of his theoretical loyalty, tends to work toward the adoption and institutionalisation of democratic procedures in small groups.

In summary, the essence of the social goals model is embodied in the words of the late Grace Coyle:

'It is not enough . . . for man to seek enjoyment in isolation from others. Because of his essentially social nature his fullest growth comes only as he uses his expanding powers in conjunction with and for the benefit of others. For his own deepest growth he must be socialized . . . we . . . mean by this his ability to establish mutual relations with others and the capacity to identify himself with the good of the social whole however he conceives it, to use his capacities in part at least for social ends beyond himself. Each must find for himself his social objects of devotion, but to discover them is as essential to fulfilment as to find the objects of his more personal loves. To hope for such attainment in however small a measure is no doubt the common goal of all who sincerely wish to work in some capacity with people.'[16]

THE REMEDIAL MODEL

Placed in historical context the remedial model further facilitated the integration of the group work method in the profession of social work. It offered a congenial base for the linkage of the social group work method with the method of social casework. As in casework, the remedial model established the treatment of individuals as the central function of group work. Through the remedial model the social group work method offered another means by which the profession could restore or rehabilitate individuals.

Early development of the remedial model was conspicuously influenced by the work of Redl in the institutional group treatment of children. Later the model was elaborated by social group workers such as Konopka, Sloan, Fisher and Gantner. A systematic formulation of the model has been presented in the writings of Robert Vinter, now identified as its major theoretician.

The problems of adjustment in personal and social relations that can be treated through the use of the group are considered within the special competence of the social group worker. Attention to such problems reaffirms 'the profession's historic mission of service to those most in need'.[15] In this manner, the concept of priority is introduced in the remedial model. Criticism is directed towards the deployment of limited personnel to those services which are categorised as 'socialisation and consumption' services.[16] It follows logically, then, that the image of the client is that of an individual who is suffering from some form of social maladaptation or deficiency. In this sense, the remedial model is clearly a clinical model focused upon helping the malperforming individual to achieve a more desirable state of social functioning.

The group is viewed as a tool or context for treatment of the individual. Diagnostic goals for each individual as established by the worker supersede group goals. '. . . changes in the group structure and the group process,' states Arthur Blum, 'are the means to the end goal of individual change. . . .'[17] Group development is not conceived in the interest of collective growth that has meaning unto itself. There is no idealised image of a healthy group *per se*. A conception of group health transcends the particular needs of the therapeutic situation. Blum continues:

'A "good" group is the group which permits and fosters the growth of its members. This does not presuppose any fixed structure or level of function as being desirable except as it affects the members. . . . Evaluation of the desirability of its [the group's] structure and processes can only be made in relation to the desirability of its effects upon the members and the potential it provides for the worker's interventions.'[18]

The treatment group primarily envisioned by the remedial model is the 'formed' group, wherein membership is predetermined and diagnostically selected by the worker.[19] Natural or friendship ties are not considered essential unless they meet the therapeutic prescription, or where there are no other bases of group formation open to the worker. Group composition is considered a significant factor in the potential of the group to serve as an effective treatment vehicle.

Processes within the group which help members to help each other are given recognition in this model but the limit of the self-help system is contained within the boundaries of the diagnostic plan. The remedial model deals only peripherally with a full range of collective associations such as are to be found in spontaneous groupings, informal lounges and mass activities. Moreover, the preventive use of the group in relation to normal developmental needs is of secondary importance. The group pro-gramme is primarily evaluated for its therapeutic potential rather than for its creative and expressive qualities.

The worker is viewed as a 'change agent' rather than an 'enabler' facilitating self-direction of the group. He uses a problem-solving approach, sequentially phasing his activities in the tradition of study, diagnosis and treatment. He is characteristically directive, and assumes a position of clinical pre-eminence and authority. He exercises this authority through such ways as the assigning of task and role, and the screening of activity against his own professional objectives. His authority derives from the mandate given to him by the profession and the agency. While his authority must be confirmed by the group, it is not fundamentally established by the group. From this position of authority his intervention may be designed to do *for* the client as well as *with* the client. The model does not require the worker to give priority to the establishment of group autonomy[20] nor to the perpetuation of the group as a self-help system.

With regard to setting, the remedial model seems to require a struc-tured institutional context. It assumes clearly defined agency policy in support of treatment goals. When these are not available, it suggests professional efforts to develop them. The remedial model makes less provision for adapting service to the informal life style of the client. It appears to depart from the tradition that the group worker engages with people where he finds them as they go about the business of daily living.

From the earliest development of the remedial model it was necessary to draw upon individual psychological theories in support of its indivi-dualising focus. The model relied heavily upon traditional sources of individual theory utilised by social casework. For example, psycho-analytic theory provided a set of concepts that sensitised the group worker to 'resistance' and 'transference' phenomena and the 'symbolic' representation of the group as a family. More recently the utility of ego psychology to explain behaviour in relation to internal and external forces is being recognised and explored.

Whereas social group work has had more difficulty operationalising psychoanalytical concepts, social role theory has lent itself to a simpler and more direct application for understanding and treating the individual in the group. The significance of this theory lies in its power to provide conceptualisations that define and describe the 'presenting' social problems more in harmony with the method of treatment to be used. Social role theory as an interactional theory, therefore, is congruent to the unit of service employed by the social group worker. It is this theory that has been employed prominently in the writings of Vinter and his colleagues at the University of Michigan School of Social Work.[21]

Since the remedial model assumes that 'group development can be controlled and influenced by the worker's actions',[22] it must draw heavily from theories of small group dynamics. These theories help to account for changes in the group and suggest opportunities for professional interventions in carrying out the 'change agent' role.

In the remedial model the central and most powerful concept is 'treatment goal'. Emphasis on this concept is intersticed throughout most of its practice principles. The influence of the 'treatment goal' is to be noted in the following selected practice principles:

(1) 'Specific treatment goals must be established for each member of the client group.'[23]
(2) The worker 'attempts to define group purposes so that they are consistent with the several treatment goals established for the individual members'.[24]
(3) The worker helps 'the group to develop that system of norms and values which is in accord with the worker's treatment goals'.[25]
(4) The worker prestructures 'the content for group sessions based on the worker's knowledge of individuals expressed through his treatment goals as well as his knowledge of structural characteristics and processes that take place within the group'.[26]

These principles state clearly that assessment begins with the needs of individual members. Knowledge of these needs is derived from information secured prior to the individual's participation in the group. It is assumed that with such knowledge the group worker can integrate individual needs into a needs-satisfying system through the formation of a group. Thus it is the group worker who diagnoses the needs and who formulates treatment goals *for the client*. The lesser emphasis on the concept *with the client* sharply differentiates the remedial model from the other two models.

The model places considerable import on possession of knowledge by the group worker as a key to diagnosis and treatment. The model assumes that (1) such knowledge is available, and (2) given the appropriate knowledge the group worker will know precisely how to act in relation to it. This is far removed from the realities of both theory and practice. Appropriate knowledge may not always be available. More often we know better from knowledge what *not* to do than what should be done. There is, in fact, a limit to prescriptiveness in the real world that is not taken into account in this model. There is a mechanistic quality about the remedial model which precludes the creative and dynamic aspects of human interaction.

A sense of unreality prevails in the demands that are made upon the group worker in the early contact with the group. In actual practice most of the group worker's initial efforts are directed toward problems of group management and maintenance in the external environment. Individual therapeutic goals are subject to the reality stress of group formation and may themselves be modified. Treatment goals during this phase provide less of an anchorage for professional activity than is implied in the model.

Further analysis of the remedial model reveals insufficient provision for a group to contribute to its environment. Actually the model constrains the group worker from viewing the group as a system to be sustained and utilised for the purpose of enhancing the milieu. 'Obviously,' says Vinter, 'the aim of group work is not to help persons to become good members of successfully operating client groups.'[27] In the remedial model the human group has little claim to existence except for what it can give to the individual. In the light of this, it is difficult to determine from this model the specificity of the group work function in contrast to the general function of group therapy. Moreover, the model leaves unanswered what is the special contribution of group work in the full spectrum of social work with groups.

Within its circumscribed boundaries, the remedial model has made several theoretical advances. It has systematically set forth (1) guidelines for diagnostic considerations of individual functioning in the group, (2) criteria for group formation, (3) foundations for clinical team participation and (4) diagnostic utilisation of the group where other treatment modalities coexist. Thus the model has greatly facilitated the functioning of group work practitioners in clinical settings, and has drawn upon the learnings from these settings for incorporation in a general framework of social group work method.

THE RECIPROCAL MODEL

This model advances a helping process that is intended to serve both the individual and society. It proceeds on the assumption that social group work is a special case of a general social work method which is addressed to the human condition whether it be presented in a single or collective context. Whereas the reciprocal model has been specifically organised by one author, William Schwartz, it reflects the influence of many contributors. It opens the way for providing a larger theoretical umbrella to encompass more adequately the whole of the social group work method.

The duality of its focus suggests Kaiser's early conceptualisation[28] in this regard. The strong emphasis on process, enabling, and on quality of engagement is reminiscent of Phillips.[29] More recently the work of Emanuel Tropp[30] illustrates possibilities of further developing several aspects of the model in greater theoretical depth.

The reciprocal model presupposes an organic, systemic relationship between the individual and society. The interdependence is described as 'symbiotic', of basic urgency to both, and normally subject to crisis and stress. This interdependence is the 'focus' for social work and the small group is the field in which individual and societal functioning can be nourished and mediated. The range of social work function can include prevention, provision, as well as restoration. Breakdown in the interdependence between systems may occur at any point on the continuum between health and pathology.

Within the logic of this model the group is in a position of pre-eminence. Since the group is accorded such central status in the model, it can be said that it is, in fact, the client of the group worker. It follows that key concepts in this model largely pertain to the group. The most striking concept of the reciprocal model is 'mutual aid system'.

Unlike the remedial model, the reciprocal model does not begin with *a priori* prescriptions or desired outcomes. However, it does conceive of an ideal group state, namely, a system in mutual aid. Such a system is not dependent upon the specific problem to be resolved by the group but is a necessary condition for problem solving. To state it in still another way, the reciprocal model has no therapeutic ends, no political or social change programme, to which it is addressed. It is only from the encounter of individuals that compose a reciprocal group system that direction or problem is determined. Emphasis is placed on *engagement* in the process of interpersonal relations. It is from this state of involvement that members may call upon each other in their own or a common cause.

Group members, states Schwartz, 'move to relate their own sense of need to the social demand implicit in the collective tasks of the group'.[31] Tropp takes this further by insisting that it is the 'common goals group . . . with shared authority . . . pursuing common decisions'[32] that is the core group at the centre of attention of the social group work method.

The concept of shared authority derives from the assumption 'that people create many helping relationships in addition to and concurrent with the one formed with the worker'.[33]

The reciprocal model views the individual primarily in terms of his motivation and capacity for reciprocity. The model, therefore, focuses on the relational aspects of behaviour as determined by the present reality of the group system. Understanding of the individual is bounded by the social context in which he, the group and the worker interact. Diagnostic considerations or structural descriptions of the individual are not regarded as significant predictors of behaviour in the group. There-fore they do not serve as a basis for selection of members for a group or assessment by the worker.

The image of the worker projected by this model is that of a mediator or enabler to the needs system converging on the group. The worker is viewed as a part of the worker–client system both influencing and being influenced by it. In the terminology of social work, he neither does *to* the client nor *for* him, but *with* him. The relationship between worker and client in this model involves deep investment and emotional com-mitment in which the worker reveals and makes available his aspirations, knowledge and effect within the boundaries of the 'contract' between himself, the group and the agency.

The reciprocal model makes no reference to a type of agency auspice, but it does assume that, whatever the agency, it will engage in the mutual establishment of a 'contract'. Thus the agency also accepts a place in a reciprocal system with inherent limitations. The authority of the agency is not emphasised in this model.

The knowledge base of the reciprocal model primarily originates in sociological systems theory and field theory. In analysing group work and constructing a formulation of group work method, a structural-functional approach is employed. However, it is to be noted that while Schwartz posits the parts-whole concept, he chooses to focus on the relationship of parts to whole, paying scant attention to the specificity or autonomy of parts themselves.

A second theoretical source, although not directly acknowledged, is implied by the reciprocal model. This theoretical source is known under the general rubric of social psychological theories of personality. Shades of Adler, Fromm and Sullivan are to be found in the assumptions that underlie the individual's motivation and capacity for reaching out to collectivities.

In turning to the practice principles generated by the reciprocal model, they are found to be first developed as generic methodology for social work as a whole and subsequently transformed for utilisation in a worker–group system.

Schwartz has conceptualised five major tasks to be carried out by the social work practitioner. In very brief form they are as follows:

(1) The task of searching out the common ground between the client's perception of his own need and the aspects of social demand with which he is faced.
(2) The task of detecting and challenging the obstacles which obscure the common ground. ...
(3) The task of contributing data – ideas, facts, value concepts – which are not available to the client. ...

(4) The task of 'lending a vision'. . . .

(5) The task of defining the requirements and the limits of the situation in which the client–worker system is set.[34]

Each of these generic tasks has been operationalised through a series of principles that specifically guides social group workers.

To illustrate, we will take task #1, that of 'searching out common ground'. The model suggests three primary principles as follows: (1) The worker helps the group to strengthen its goals through a consideration of what it is in common that the members are seeking. (2) The worker interprets his role through clarifying with the group what it is they wish from him that he has available to give, from which a clear 'contractual' agreement can be drawn. (3) The worker acts to protect the focus of work against attempts to evade or subvert it.

Pervading this model is a series of practice principles that are devoted to worker honesty and directness and the avoidance of withholding knowledge and effect. These principles seem to reflect as much the author's determination to dispel a 'mystique of professionalism' as to relate to the functional tasks

The contribution of the reciprocal model lies in its unifying abstractions. Intensive individualising and social focusing within the small group are rendered in a conceptual balance, providing a coherent footing for further theoretical development.

The limitation of Schwartz's formulation lies more in theoretical *gaps* than in inconsistencies. Middle-range supporting theories are insufficiently developed in several areas. For example, interest in the individual system is strikingly sparse. Schwartz does not make allowance for the latitude of human personality which may be necessary to explain the manner in which the individual coheres in any system in aid of others. There is a sense of unreality in the notion that the motivation toward collectivity is always productive of individual and/or social good. Without guidelines in relation to individual dynamics and normative expectations, there is no basis for assessing the impact of change upon individuals. There is produced a tendency toward permissiveness and abdication of worker's authority. Process itself is elevated to an unreal superordinance.

It is to be noted that ego-psychological concepts increasingly being utilised by social group workers may fill the gap regarding individual dynamics without violating the central logic of the reciprocal model.[35]

Group system theory is likewise underdeveloped. Schwartz does not sufficiently take into account similarities or differences in a variety of group systems. Moreover, while his conceptualisation is useful in beginning with a group, it does not offer a framework for dealing with changes that may occur in the group over time. Thus the model ignores what has

been observed experientially by group workers and is known from scientific study of small groups. Group development is perceived simplistic-
ally, without conceptually accounting for new levels realisable as a result
of group experience and achievement.

Schwartz's formulation is distressingly lacking in any clarification of
group programme. One might deduce that discussion as a channel for
communication overshadows all others.

It seems appropriate now to recall Irving Miller's comments on an
earlier form of this paper. He addressed himself to the level of abstraction of a theoretical model. He raised the possibility that 'the concrete
solutions and specific applications which may be eventually deduced
from a broad and generalised model may be so attenuated as to suggest
that the specific applications do not necessarily flow from or require the
original abstraction'.[36]

Despite limitations of the reciprocal model, its outstanding contribution is the construct of a mutual aid system with professional interventions flowing from it. What has been vaguely referred to in the past
as 'helping members to help themselves' has acquired a higher level of
theoretical statement. It is possible now to consider systematically the
attributes and culture of such a specialised system and to transmit the
skills necessary to support its realisation. This is probably the single
most important contribution that group work method can make to the
social work profession at large.

In conclusion, we submit that the significant movement of social group
work in theory building lies in the production of models systematic
designs by which the elements of social group work practice have begun
to be ordered and problems in practice rendered more solvable. We
have found three models to be clearly in existence. Each independently
pursues lines of inquiry relating historical tradition to present societal
requirements. The foremost contribution of each is not made by the
other two. Each falls short in encompassing the totality of social group
work method. This suggests that new models will emerge either parallel
or in a subsuming relationship to those that presently exist.

Even as the kinship of all social group workers to each of these
models insists itself upon us, so also the continued authorship of our
theory lies with each of us. Regardless of the particular bias of practice
or educational institution, it is essential that all new practitioners enter
the profession with a knowledge of the state of its theoretical development and with ability to relate their thinking to the models that exist.

Furthermore, all practitioners and educators writing today about social
group work practice should in some manner take into account where
their work falls in relation to these patternings that have developed.
Thus each of these models will be moved ahead in order, fullness and
complexity or will be replaced by more useful theoretical structures.

The possession of models provides a baseline for further elaborating the utility of the social group work method in the profession's service to mankind.

NOTES AND REFERENCES FOR CHAPTER 8

1 Leonard S. Kogan, 'Principles of measurement', in Norman A. Polansky (ed.), *Social Work Research* (Chicago: University of Chicago Press, 1960), p. 90.
2 The formulation of this analytical frame borrows heavily from Robert D. Vinter, 'Problems and processes in developing group work practice principles', *Theory Building in Social Work*, Workshop Report, CSWE 1960 Annual Program Meeting (New York: Council on Social Work Education, 1960).
3 Mildred Sirls *et al.*, *Social Group Practice Elaborated: A Statement of Position* (Pittsburgh: University of Pittsburgh Graduate School of Social Work, April 1964; mimeographed).
4 Hyman J. Wiener, 'Social change and social group work practice', *Social Work*, vol. IX, no. 3 (July 1964).
5 Mitchell I. Ginsberg and Jack R. Goldberg, 'The impact of the current scene on group work policy and practice', *Summary Presentations: Group Work Section Meetings, 1961–1962*, p. 30.
6 Joseph D. Jacobs, 'Social action as therapy in a mental hospital', *Social Work*, vol. IX, no. 1 (January 1964).
7 Wiener, 'Social change and social group work practice', p. 109.
8 ibid.
9 ibid.
10 ibid.
11 ibid.
12 Eleanor L. Ryder, 'Some principles of intergroup relations as applied to group work', *Social Work With Groups 1960* (New York: National Association of Social Workers, 1960), pp. 52–61.
13 Jack Wiener, 'Reducing racial and religious discrimination', *Social Work With Groups 1960* (New York: National Association of Social Workers, 1960), pp. 62–73.
14 Grace L. Coyle, *Group Work with American Youth* (New York: Harper & Brothers, 1948).
15 Robert D. Vinter, 'Group work: perspectives and prospects', *Social Work With Groups 1959* (New York: National Association of Social Workers, 1959), p. 135.
16 ibid., p. 136.
17 Arthur Blum, 'The social group work method: one view', *A Conceptual Framework for the Teaching of the Social Group Work Method in the Classroom* (New York: Council on Social Work Education, 1964), p. 12.
18 loc. cit.
19 For further amplification see Rosemary Sarri *et al.*, *Diagnosis in Social Group Work* (Ann Arbor: University of Michigan School of Social Work, October 1964; mimeographed).
20 This same observation was made by Mildred Sirls *et al.*, *Social Group Practice Elaborated*, p. 6.
21 For elaboration on the use of social role theory in group work practice, see Paul H. Glasser, 'Social role, personality, and group work practice', *Social Work Practice* (New York: Columbia University Press, 1962), pp. 60–74.
22 Rosemary C. Sarri and Maeda J. Galinsky, 'A conceptual framework for

teaching group development in social group work', *A Conceptual Framework for the Teaching of the Social Group Work Method in the Classroom* (New York: Council on Social Work Education, 1964), p. 21.

23 Robert D. Vinter, 'The essential components of social group work practice' (Ann Arbor: University of Michigan School of Social Work, 1959), p. 4 (mimeographed).

24 ibid., p. 6.

25 ibid., p. 12.

26 Paul H. Glasser and Jane Costabile, 'Social group work practice in a public welfare setting' (Ann Arbor: University of Michigan School of Social Work, November 1963), p. 4 (mimeographed).

27 Robert D. Vinter, 'The essential components of social group work practice', p. 6.

28 Clara Kaiser, 'The social group work process', *Journal of Social Work* (April 1958), pp. 67–75.

29 Helen Phillips, *Essentials of Social Group Work Skill* (New York: Association Press, 1957).

30 Emanuel Tropp, 'Group intent and group structure: essential criteria for group work practice', *Journal of Jewish Communal Service*, vol. XLI, no. 3 (Spring 1965).

31 William Schwartz, 'Toward a strategy of group work practice', *Social Service Review* (September 1962), p. 274.

32 Tropp, 'Group intent and group structure', p. 234.

33 Schwartz, 'Toward a strategy of group work practice', p. 273.

34 William Schwartz, 'The social worker in the group', *New Perspectives on Services to Groups* (New York: National Association of Social Workers, 1961), p. 17.

35 A most current example is to be found in Baruch Levine, 'Principles for developing an ego supportive group treatment service', *Social Service Review*, vol. XXXIV, no. 4 (December 1965).

36 The original form of this paper was presented at Columbia University School of Social Work Alumni Conference, April 1962. Irving Miller served as a discussant.

Chapter 9

SOCIAL GROUP WORK IN THE UNITED KINGDOM

Nano McCaughan

Social group work originated as a social work method in a variety of social movements over the last hundred years. Its development has been supported and enriched by theoretical developments in the behavioural sciences which provide knowledge about the nature and growth of man and about the effects of different means used for the solution of social problems. To understand the functions and philosophy of the social group work method it will be useful to review some of these major ideas.

During the nineteenth century, several movements sponsored the formation of clubs and associations for the socially deprived. Most of these movements were based on the belief that social reform would be brought about by associations of people who joined together for mutual aid. An example of such movements is the settlement house organisation. Settlement houses were established in deprived working-class inner-city areas, and staffed by university graduates. Canon Barnett, the founder of the first settlement at Toynbee Hall, stated that his objective was for settlement residents 'to form friendships [with local people] and then through friendship to raise the standard of living and of life'.[1] Settlement workers facilitated the formation of groups with spiritual, educational and cultural purposes.

During the same period there were developed many self-help, co-operative and mutual aid societies. The co-operative movement started with the objective of providing the means for the democratic production and distribution of food. Though there was a strong economic element in its origin, the movement soon expanded its purposes to provide educational and leisure-time opportunities for mothers and, perhaps more importantly, to provide opportunities for the poor to develop leadership in local groups.

Octavia Hill's work with housing estates included significant work with groups. For example, on the housing estate that she managed she sponsored the formation of play groups, mothers' groups and even a fathers' group.

These nineteenth-century movements accepted the dual purpose inherent in group membership: social action for the benefit of the group and individual enrichment through the sense of belonging and the opportunity to befriend and assist others. Although these efforts often stemmed from a desire to further Christian beliefs and practices or (as in the case of the settlement and many similar organisations) to inculcate middle-class values in working-class areas, they attempted also to train indigenous members of the population in civic responsibility and leadership.

Throughout the twentieth century there has been a proliferation of social movements, many of the objectives of which constitute the basis for social work practice today. For example, among the many youth organisations that have the objectives of 'rescue', recreation and provision of resources, there are some, such as the scouting movement, that make effective use of small groups in their work.

The development of social group work occurred in a similar fashion in the United States with close connections between social reform and social work via the group method. For example, during the 1920s a group of practitioners and researchers met together in New York City to study the activities and development of social agencies that provided leisure and recreational opportunities for the young and poor. This group became known by the title of their journal, *The Inquiry*. Their aim was to understand how group processes could be utilised for effective citizenship and to counteract the worst features of bureaucracy.

Grace Coyle, one of the outstanding figures associated with *The Inquiry*, became the link between practitioners and researchers. Using concepts from both sociology and psychology, the group began to develop a theoretical base for the practice of social group work. These concepts illuminated the processes of group learning and decision making and moved the emphasis away from activities. Shortly afterwards, in 1926, Grace Coyle initiated the first training programme for social group workers at the School of Applied Social Sciences, Western Reserve University, Cleveland, Ohio.

Up to that time, training for social group work was based on the social goals model as it is described by Papell and Rothman.[2] Essentially, through the 1920s the major goals of group work were concerned with social action and citizenship training and with the inculcation of leadership skills in indigenous members. Subsequent development in the use of the group as a medium for individual change and growth stemmed from group therapy techniques which originated in work with the psychologically-damaged servicemen of the Second World War.

In the United Kingdom, W. R. Bion[3] and his colleagues at the Tavistock Institute of Human Relations, using the ideas of Freud[4] and Melanie Klein,[5] formulated psychological propositions about group behaviour, focusing particularly on attitudes towards authority and intimacy. The work has been expanded at the Tavistock Institute, the Grubb Institute of Behavioural Studies, the Institute of Group Analysis and others in studies of organisational behaviour and the effects of environmental systems that impinge on the group. In their work with groups, many British social workers have been influenced by training programmes that evolved from these developments. However, it is difficult for some to integrate 'learning through experiencing' via their own participation in groups with the more cognitive learning required to master an ever-increasing body of knowledge from sociological and psychological research on small groups.

In the United Kingdom the development of social group work (as distinct from 'group psycho-therapy') has lagged behind the United States. It was first given official recognition by the Youth Service which was created by the Ministry of Education during the Second World War to provide facilities for leisure time and informal education. Courses on group work were offered in the training programmes for youth and community workers that were developed to train workers for these services. But as late as 1960 the Albemarle Report[6] called for better training facilities and implied that teaching for group work was inadequate.

Until recently, training for work with groups has been almost completely absent in social work training courses. In 1958, the Younghusband Report[7] described group work as a form of social work practice that provides constructive group experiences that enable people to develop as individuals and to contribute to the life of the community. The Report noted that very little teaching about group processes or interventive skills was offered on professional social work courses at that time. The Report also pointed to the desirability of using group work skills in centres for the handicapped, clubs for the disabled, temporary accommodation for the homeless, hostels and residential institutions, and in the work of home help organisers. The Report identified an important dimension of social work with groups, namely that different and specific aims, purposes and methods should be developed for different settings.

However, almost ten years later, in the Report of the Seebohm Committee[8] little attention is devoted to group work except to echo Younghusband in stating that 'Social workers are more and more concerned with the whole family as a group and also find themselves with other clients in groups'. Seebohm does not carry the idea farther. For example, there is no suggestion that social work in the social services should develop and encourage the deliberate formation of client groups for the purpose of individual enrichment, treatment and change, as well as for social action.

Group work has been demonstrated to be an effective mode of intervention in enabling some types of clients to solve social problems. Evidence for this has been produced in such studies as the Wincroft Youth

Project,[9] the Canford Families[10] and the (unanticipated) findings of 'Girls at Vocational High'[11] respecting the effects of group experience. In the last ten years, despite difficulties presented by the dearth of field-work training experiences and insufficient teaching about group processes, there has been an increasing use of group methods in the work of the probation service, prisons, voluntary social agencies and in social service departments. Some of the impetus for these developments may well have come from the ever-increasing number of 'self-help' groups that seem to be effective in achieving therapeutic and social objectives such as Alcoholics Anonymous, Synanon, Claimants Union and the Preservation of the Rights of Prisoners (PROP).

Another important influence has come from work in therapeutic communities with mentally ill adults and maladjusted children. Here the total staff-resident group has been viewed as a medium of therapy and change.[12]

OBJECTIVES IN GROUP WORK

These various strands in the use of groups have led to a wide variation in the conceptualisation of objectives, processes and tasks in work with groups. A variety of models are available for practitioners to use in organising their work. In the following paragraphs we will describe group work in terms of different types of objectives, targets, worker roles and timing. Broadly speaking, groups may be organised for the purpose of enabling clients to attain goals that can be categorised along a continuum ranging from intrapsychic, interpersonal, inter-environmental to inter-group. These types of groups are 'ideal types'. In fact, most groups operate with some mixture of objectives. The usefulness of the classification lies mainly in the attempt to clarify the varying goals groups may pursue through different phases and the implications these objectives have for direction and organisation. We can identify these varying objectives as follows:

(1) *Group work to enable individuals to achieve some inner personality change or adjustment that will enhance their functioning in a variety of social roles such as parent, spouse, worker and friend.* An example of group work based on this objective is a group run by a social worker (sometimes with a psychiatrist as co-therapist) for young psychiatric in-patients suffering from personality or mood disorders. Other examples are work with groups to enable members to solve specific problems that interfere with their performance in an important social role, and with groups of newly-disabled men who need help in accepting their residual disability and finding appropriate employment. These group experiences involve some relearning or readjustment to familiar role performances. The emphasis in these groups is on therapy and restoration.

(2) *Group work to enable individuals to take on new roles.* With this objective group experiences are utilised to help people prepare for a reasonably common but stressful life event such as entering an institution and adopting a child. A variant of this is group work with the objective of enabling members to take on social caring roles, such as with a group of adults who are preparing to become foster parents. The emphasis in groups of this kind is on education and prevention.

(3) *Groups that provide individuals with missing life experiences by the provision of physical and emotional resources.* The aim here is to bring about enhanced interpersonal relations among the members by

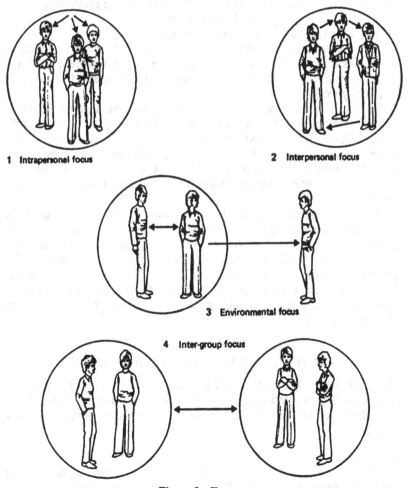

1 Intrapersonal focus   2 Interpersonal focus

3 Environmental focus

4 Inter-group focus

Figure 2   Targets

means of group experience. This goal is often referred to as 'psychological growth' or 'increased maturity'. It is expected that the provision of missing resources will enable participants to expand their capacities to utilise resources in their community, families, schools, work groups, and so forth. An example would be a group for socially and economically deprived young people. The emphasis in this group is on social learning in the 'here and now'.

(4) *Group work with the objective of improving communication or reciprocal transactions between two systems.* An example is work with a Parent–Teacher Association and a school over a common problem like truancy, or with a group of psychiatric in-patients and their ward staff focusing on questions of policy or group relations. The emphasis in these groups is on developing social consciousness.

These four types are illustrated in Figure 2.

There are two other types of group work that have not been included in our classification. At this point in time they appear to be the subject of boundary disputes between workers with individuals and families, and community workers.

The first of these types is work with the family as a group, which is rapidly developing a theory and body of knowledge of its own with concepts drawn from individual psychology, communications theory and group dynamics.[18] Other 'natural' groups, such as neighbours and members of a residential community, would most easily be thought about in terms of intervention with the objectives described above as types 2, 3 and 4.

The other type of group work not included in our typology is of the genre wherein social action is expressly emphasised as a goal from the group's inception. Social action is often considered to be the end result of social group work or as part of the interventive 'programme' for members. In this kind of work the professional assumes that the objective of individual enrichment and personal development must be complemented by the aim of acquiring resources for the group or a section of the community.

TARGETS, WORKER ROLES AND TIMING

There are many characteristics of practice that vary with the four types of objectives mentioned and we shall give only three as examples. These are: target of change, worker roles and techniques, and length and timing.

(1) Targets
With interpersonal and intrapersonal types of change objectives, the target of change is primarily the inner world of the members whether

the change is to enable members to overcome specific problems or to alter existing attitudinal and behavioural patterns. This has implications for group composition. Groups of this type should be composed of individuals who have undergone a diagnostic screening. The search for commonality with others is conducted *before* the group commences. Because of the high degree of discretion and authority that rests with the worker regarding group composition and selection of members, these types of groups are appropriately referred to as 'artificial'.

In groups with an environmental focus the target of change tends to be the group itself; members are recruited from a loosely defined category such as 'deprived children' or 'isolated mothers' in a neighbourhood. The members may also constitute a 'natural group' such as a street-corner gang, or a ward of patients in a mental hospital. The search for commonality of goal is seen as an important learning experience and takes place after the group is under way.

Groups with an inter-group focus by definition require that the work is carried on with 'natural' groups in which people are already involved in reciprocal interaction with others. The focus of change is the interaction between groups which, in Schwartz's view, is the 'encounter between the individual and his society'.[14]

(2) Worker Roles

The worker's role relationships with members will vary considerably according to group objectives. In groups with an intrapersonal focus he takes on the role of 'expert' in human functioning, using his professional knowledge to assist members to solve problems under his direction. As Papell and Rothman state, his authority stems from his profession and from his agency's objectives as well as from the mandate given to him by his clients.[15] The methods of work are likely to include a good deal of discussion and analysis of feelings and actions; increasingly, techniques such as role play and behaviour rehearsal are used. This type of work is, approximately, what is described by R. Vinter and his colleagues.[16]

In groups with an interpersonal and environmental focus the worker attempts to fulfil the role of enabler; he works to create a 'mutual aid system', to borrow Professor Schwartz's phrase, and he perceives the members as his working partners. He acts on the assumption that the member's pool of experience is greater than his own. In the role of enabler or facilitator his tasks are defined mainly in terms of attempting to create an open and effective communication system within the group. The mandate for his authority comes primarily from the group members. The techniques used in these types of group work include discussion, debate, and a variety of task and recreational activities in the performance of which people relate to one another.

Activities include painting, games, socio-drama, provision and cooking of food, dressmaking and decision-making exercises. Selection of activities depends on the age range and social problems of the members. The activities are used in a thoughtful way, with consideration of both their latent and manifest efforts. For example, in working with a group of over-active, aggressive children, a worker would plan for the introduction of games to relieve bodily tensions, to produce appropriate aggression in timid members and to produce co-operative activity. He would try to provide opportunities for all members to assume a variety of roles and introduce activities in which even the least competent could succeed.

The worker tends to be 'closer' to members in these types of groups. He might take the opportunity to drive them home or to go with them on an outing for social or recreational purposes. He encourages familiarity and he believes that it is enabling to share his own life experiences and problems. A major difficulty that he faces is doing this while at the same time remaining sufficiently on the boundaries of the group to help members become more sensitive to and learn from the experiences they are sharing.

In groups with an inter-group focus the worker's role is to serve as an intermediary between two groups. Although he may be perceived by one or the other, or both, as an ally or an enemy, his intellectual task is to understand the structure and dynamics of two systems in conflict. These tasks require that he help the client system to organise and to reach a consensus in defining their problems in relation to another system. This may involve, for example, the creation of a committee-type structure with leadership in the hands of members. In work with an institutional agency system the worker will try to enable members of that agency (e.g. professional social welfare workers) to understand the discrepancy between its manifest and its latent objectives in work with client systems. He will often undertake a considerable amount of work with individuals in these systems.

(3) Timing

In groups that have the goal of intra-psychic change, the work will be intensive with weekly or bi-weekly meetings. Such groups usually last for at least one year and sometimes continue for up to five years. Group work with individuals preparing to take on a new role tends to be intensive but short term. Sometimes the objective may be attained in four to eight group sessions. Growth-oriented groups also tend to be long term and the timing of contact will vary. They sometimes include a period of residential living such as a camping holiday. These groups vary as to whether they are 'open' or 'closed' systems. Some groups may be composed of the same individuals while in other groups members may leave and new members may be introduced. In groups with an inter-group focus the work continues until the defined problems are ameliorated or solved and this may require anything from a few days to several months.

KNOWLEDGE SPECIFIC TO GROUP WORK

Papell and Rothman outline three different models of group work practice for which they describe the different emphases regarding the knowledge utilised, the target system and the worker's roles and tasks. In the absence of empirical knowledge about the relative effectiveness of these models for solving problems, it is important that group workers identify the knowledge they require to develop skill in practice. The model that a worker selects for practice should be relevant to the purpose of the group with which he works. For example, with the objective of helping people solve a specific problem or prepare themselves for a new role, the remedial model, as explicated by Vinter,[17] would be the most appropriate one. The objectives of promoting personal growth and providing groups with leisure resources might draw on the social goals model developed in the writings of Phillips,[18] Konopka[19] and Bernstein.[20] For the objective of using groups for mediation, the work of Schwartz[21] would be most useful.

Some areas of knowledge about human behaviour and societal functioning are common to all models of social group work. This common knowledge includes the following: (1) knowledge about group life and its significance for the development of individuals and societies in both fulfilling and frustrating instinctual, social and economic needs; (2) knowledge about communication processes and transactions among people, utilising concepts from role therapy, group dynamics and transactional analysis; (3) knowledge about group decision-making processes and about power and influence in small groups; (4) knowledge about how groups develop over time including the stages in the life of groups, the needs and problems that arise in different stages, and the varying models of leadership that are effective at different stages; and (5) knowledge about inter-group relations, the processes of labelling people deviant, and the problems encountered in representing one group to another.

This kind of knowledge is acquired both cognitively and emotionally. Training programmes should be devised to offer learning from experience coupled with analytic reflection.

Knowledge for group work practice can be described in terms of the worker's tasks in the different phases of group development. These tasks include:

(1) *Composing a viable group* or integrating oneself with an already formed one; involving members in articulating common problems

and achieving agreement on paths to follow towards selected goals; making a contract with the group as to how long it will exist and whether it is to be an 'open' or 'closed' system.

(2) *Guiding the development of a clear and authentic communication system*, avoiding the pitfalls of false consensus; *providing leadership* through self or others; *offering reinforcement* to activities that are goal directed and, by question and clarification, helping the group deal with those that are not.

(3) *Identifying and helping the group acquire resources* needed for the continuance of the group.

(4) *Involving the group in the selection of appropriate problem-solving methods* such as using non-verbal or verbal activities. This requires an assessment of the opportunities offered by the group for individuals to rethink attitudes and to learn new social skills, and to acquire competence in dealing with other systems by doing, by discussion and by the development of cognitive awareness.

(5) *Analysing the continuing group situation, judging its developmental level* and current aspirations and *enabling individuals to express ideas* from which the group can work out modified objectives.

(6) *Enabling the group to recognise the limits placed on it by other groups* and supporting the group in its efforts to adapt to these limits or to alter them.

(7) *Monitoring group organisation and structure to ensure that roles do not become fixed* and that each individual finds a place in the group and is offered a variety of roles over time.

(8) *Terminating the work* for an individual or the group; involving the group in the evaluation process and *enabling individuals to deal with separation* as constructively as possible.

(9) *Recording the group's progress* and using records both for service to the group and for professional development.

CURRENT ISSUES AND PROBLEMS IN SOCIAL GROUP WORK

One of the difficulties in developing an integrated approach to social work methods in the United Kingdom is the current lack of skills and knowledge in the use of group methods. This deficiency is due, in part, to the separation of training for youth and community work (which, at this time, is the responsibility of the Department of Education and Science) from training for social work. For many years the only exposure that most social workers had to group work was the therapy groups run by psychiatrists using depth-counselling techniques. Working with groups for other purposes such as recreation and training in social skills has been regarded as unnecessary for social workers. Some social workers (particularly older, more experienced workers in positions of seniority) consider group work to be a dangerous tool in the hands of anyone but qualified group psycho-therapists. They may be influenced in this view by an anxiety-provoking experience in a sensitivity group, coupled with insufficient opportunity to conceptualise and add to this experience from a systematic study of small group theory and social group work methods. Alternatively, they may regard group work as an alien method, particularly if it involves use of games, arts and craft activities, teaching of housewifery skills and other non-verbal aids to interpersonal change that are unfamiliar to the practice of casework.

From a theoretical point of view there are still unresolved problems relating to the integration of diverse pieces of knowledge gained from research and observation of groups. For example, many research findings are based on the study of short-term, artificially composed small groups. It may be unwise to apply conclusions drawn from the behaviour of laboratory groups to natural groups which operate over longer periods of time. Toren[22] points out that the contrived group is detached from everyday life experiences and the community norms and controls that the natural group experiences.

Another problem for group workers is the choice of appropriate models of practice. As Papell and Rothman point out, models of practice are based on differing ideas about the functions of social work, the nature of man and the dynamics of individual and social change. Models vary in degrees of conceptual specificity. The Vinter model is easier to communicate and teach, for example, than that propounded by Schwartz. As yet there is no appropriate model for those who, in order to intensify the group's learning or to enable it to deal effectively with another system, might seek to generate group conflict rather than develop a consensus approach.

As Rosenthal points out, group workers have to use two kinds of theory: *prescriptive theory* is used in the design, formation and maintenance of a group and *descriptive theory* is used in the observation of the group, the behaviour of the worker and the impinging environment.[23] Rosenthal quotes an educationalist's definition: '*Prescriptive* theory describes what ought to be done or thought. . . . The prescriptive theorist is applying knowledge: he is not seeking it . . . men who create *descriptive* theories are seeking to discover knowledge which they do not possess'. Many statements found in group work texts consist of a confusing commingling of these two kinds of theory. For example, theories about the stages of group development often seem to contain a mixture of statements about what *ought* to happen in all small groups and what *does* happen in some. In practice the strain of working with both kinds of theory can lead to inconsistent role behaviour on the part of the worker as he moves, in his imagination, from the centre (controller) of the group to the boundary (observer).

For these and other reasons there has not been a systematic development of the social group work method and only in rare instances are clients offered a choice between group or individual treatment. There has been little opportunity to study and test different forms of group treatment.

In spite of these problems, social group work is at last beginning to find its place in the repertoire of social work interventions. With the increasing problems caused by social isolation and alienation, group work can be a useful substitute for the vanishing mutual aid systems of the extended family and closely knit neighbourhoods. In certain situations groups can be a more powerful instrument for change than a relationship with an individual. Sometimes, clients working as a group make demands on the agency or some other institution to which the agency is related. These demands may be perceived as awkward or excessive. In such instances, the social worker who represents both the agency's goals and the group's goals can be in a difficult position. However, these kinds of interaction can help the agency to become more responsive to the needs and attitudes of its consumers. Hopefully, with further research and evaluation, advances will be made in our knowledge about the effectiveness of different types of groups and programmes in enabling clients to deal with their environments and to work creatively at their problems.

NOTES AND REFERENCES FOR CHAPTER 9

1 Pamphlet written by Barnett in 1869 quoted in P. Seed, *The Expansion of Social Work in Great Britain* (London: Routledge & Kegan Paul, 1973), p. 33.
2 See Chapter 8 of this volume.
3 W. R. Bion, *Experiences in Groups* (London: Tavistock Publications, 1961).
4 S. Freud, *Group Psychology and Analysis of the Ego* (London: Hogarth, 1959).
5 See, for example, *Our Adult World and Other Essays* (Bath: Pitman Press, 1963).
6 *Report on the Youth Service in England and Wales* (London: HMSO, 1960).
7 *Report of the Working Party on Social Workers*, paras 629 and 638.
8 *Report of the Committee on Local Authority and Allied Personal Social Services*, para. 556.
9 C. S. Smith, M. R. Farrant and H. J. Marchant, *Wincroft Youth Project* (London: Tavistock, 1972).
10 Paul Halmos (ed.), *Sociological Review Monograph* no. 6, 'Canford Families' (Keele: University of Keele, 1962).
11 Henry J. Meyer, *Girls at Vocational High* (New York: Russell Sage Foundation, 1965).
12 See, for example, Maxwell Jones *et al.*, *Social Psychiatry: A Study of Therapeutic Communities* (London: Tavistock, 1952).

13 See Virginia Satir, *Conjoint Family Therapy* (California: Science and Behaviour Books, 1967).
14 W. Schwartz and S. Zalba, *The Practice of Group Work* (New York: University of Columbia Press, 1971), p. 6.
15 See Chapter 8 of this volume.
16 Vinter, 'The essential components of social group work practice', in *Readings in Group Work Practice*, pp. 8–39.
17 ibid.
18 Helen Phillips, *Essentials of Social Group Work Skills* (New York: Association Press, 1959).
19 Gisela Konopka, *Social Group Work: A Helping Process* (Englewood Cliffs, NJ: Prentice-Hall, 1963).
20 Saul Bernstein (ed.), *Explorations in Group Work* and *Further Explorations in Group Work* (London: Bookstall Publications, 1973).
21 See Schwartz and Zalba, *The Practice of Group Work*.
22 N. Toren, *Social Work: The Case of a Semi-Profession* (New York: Sage Publications, 1973), pp. 208–12.
23 W. A. Rosenthal, 'Social group work theory', *Social Work* (NY), vol. XVIII, no. 5 (September 1973), pp. 60–6.

Chapter 10

COMMUNITY WORK IN THE UNITED KINGDOM*

David Jones

Community work embraces a wide and varied range of purposes and tasks and is a developing feature of a number of different services and professional activities.

The initial discussion of the Seebohm Report focused almost entirely on the problems of integrating previously separated services. Faced with escalating demand, social service departments have inevitably been preoccupied with issues of resources and internal organisation. Less attention has been given to their external relations with other agencies and with the communities they serve. Yet the development of external relations is crucial to the future quality, quantity and appropriateness of the services. The Seebohm Committee's recommendations in this connection are the most innovative and potentially far-reaching of the entire Report. The strategy sketched for the personal social services by the Seebohm Committee requires for its implementation a range of organising and planning activities, currently rather vaguely labelled 'community work'.

This paper provides an overview of community work within the context of social work. Before describing community work it may, however, be useful to review some popular conceptions of the field and to recapitulate briefly its historical development.

WHAT IS NOT COMMUNITY WORK?

People often talk as though any kind of helping activity or service is community work. But an activity is even more likely to be considered community work if it is provided off the agency's premises; if the enterprise is under non-statutory auspices; and if it involves volunteers, especially young volunteers who are more 'community' than other volunteers.

Much of what is identified as community work in this loose way may be very desirable in its own right and, in appropriate circumstances,

* Revised version of mimeograph paper (NISW, 1967).

community work may have these characteristics. But to use the term community work so broadly is pointless. It also confuses discussion in that it identifies the activity by selecting some of the characteristics frequently associated with it rather than the characteristics of the activity itself.

The term 'community work' is also sometimes used synonymously with the notion of 'community care'. A major trend in the last ten years has been the shift in emphasis from institutional care to community care. This emphasis involves the provision of an increasing range of supportive services to people in their own home situation thus enabling the handicapped, the aged, the physically ill, the mentally disordered, delinquents, neglected children, and so on either to stay in their own milieu or, if they have to leave it, to enable them to return to it as soon as possible. Increasingly, with a whole range of disabilities and problems, the period away from home and family, if it proves necessary at all, is no longer regarded as a solution or as a self-contained episode but merely as a phase in a process that starts well before the person goes away; and this process continues during the period of absence and until after he returns home.

However, caring for people in the community as contrasted with institutional care is not community work. Community work can make an important contribution to the development of community care services just as it can to the development of residential care. Thus, while development of community care services logically requires the use of community work methods, community care and community work are not synonymous.

Finally, community work is sometimes talked about as though it is an alternative to casework or as a new approach that is going to take over from casework. This idea, like some other popular conceptions of community work, is mistaken. Community work may obviate or reduce some of the problems with which caseworkers are expected to deal. For some problems, community work is a much more appropriate response than casework But there are some problems for which casework is the method of choice. Rather than reducing the need for casework, community work is more likely to increase the demand for casework services. And, hopefully, it is likely to ensure the more appropriate deployment of casework resources.

Community work may also contribute to an enlarged conception of casework. Casework along with many other helping activities in such fields as medicine, education, housing and planning needs to develop a community orientation. While all individual helping services may need to become more family and community oriented, it does not follow that caseworkers should become community workers, only that they be better caseworkers.

WHO IS NOT A COMMUNITY WORKER?

In recent years, social workers and others working in the social services have become increasingly concerned with collective social problems and questions of social policy. As citizens they have become involved in social action on matters affecting them personally; as employees they have become concerned with modifying and developing the practices and policies of the agencies in which they work; as members of professional associations they are attempting to make an impact on social policy.

These are all perfectly appropriate and desirable activities and relevant to the consideration of community work. But to regard them as the equivalent of community work merely confuses the matter.

People in a variety of positions – from publicans to policemen, from company directors to caretakers – may on occasion, either intentionally or spontaneously, act as community change agents. While this activity may be socially useful and desirable, it is not the case that such activity makes them community workers.

A further distinction relates to certain people whose activities in terms of processes, methods, techniques and objectives have much in common with community work but who nevertheless need to be distinguished from community workers in a social work context. I am thinking of organisers of social movements of various kinds. Such people may engage in the same kinds of processes as social work community workers. Indeed, in some cases it is hard to draw any sharp dividing line. But for the purposes of discussion it is necessary to make a distinction, not in terms of the desirability of the activities, but in terms of the position of the worker in relation to the issues involved and to the people being worked with. To exaggerate the distinction: the movement organiser is personally committed to the specific objectives being pursued, adopts a leadership position in relation to those being worked with and sees the individuals and groups being organised as instrumental to his own or his group's purposes. The community worker in a social work context is not necessarily personally committed to the specific objectives, adopts an enabling, supporting role rather than a leadership one and sees the individuals and groups being organised as ends rather than means.

HISTORICAL ANTECEDENTS

Social work interest in community work is a relatively new phenomenon but the ideas involved can be traced back a long way and to a variety of sources.

In 1959 the Younghusband Report stated that there are three social work methods: work with individuals (casework), groups (group work) and communities (community organisation). We can rightly point to our own indigenous tradition of social reform which goes back well into the nineteenth century as manifest in settlements, co-ordination of social services (e.g. the Charity Organisation Society recently celebrated its centenary), adult education, mutual aid movements such as the Friendly Societies, the co-operative movement and the trade unions, and a scientific approach to social problems as exemplified by the work of Charles Booth. However, the formulation of social work in terms of casework, group work and community organisation clearly reflects experience and thinking in the USA.

This threefold categorisation of social work has become more or less part of the folklore of social work in this country so it may be useful to make some distinctions between Britain and the US in this regard.

CASEWORK

In the post-1948 years, social work in Britain was equated largely with casework. There are many definitions and views of casework. The definition provided by the Younghusband Report is representative of the thinking of a majority of casework practitioners:

> 'Casework is a *personal* service provided by qualified workers for *individuals* who require skilled assistance in resolving some material, emotional or character problem. It is a disciplined activity which requires a full appreciation of the needs of the client in his family and community setting. The caseworker asks to perform this service on the basis of mutual trust and in such ways as will strengthen the client's own capacities to deal with his problems to achieve a *better adjustment with his environment*. The services required of a case-worker cover many kinds of human need, ranging from relatively simple problems of material assistance to complex personal situations involving emotional disturbance or a character deficit, which may require prolonged assistance and the careful *mobilisation of resources* and different professional skills.'[1]

This definition makes it clear that casework is concerned with social as well as personal factors; with the adjustment of the environment as well as the individual; with mobilising community resources as well as personal resources. There is, too, the implicit assumption in the practice of casework that it benefits not only the individual but society. The betterment of society, however, follows from the betterment of the individual and casework is concerned primarily with the development and adjustment of the individual rather than with societal arrangements in any general sense.

GROUP WORK

Group work has been more highly developed as a method in the USA than in this country. A fairly representative American definition reads:

> 'Social group work is a method through which individuals in groups in social agency settings are helped by a worker who guides their interaction in program activities so that they may relate themselves to others and experience growth opportunities in accordance with their needs and capacities to the end of individual, group and community development.
>
> 'In social group work, the group itself is utilised by the individual, with the help of the worker as a primary means of personality growth, change and development. The worker is interested in helping to bring about individual growth and social development for the group as a whole and for the community as a result of guided group interaction.'[2]

This perhaps gives a reasonably concrete idea of group work. Here too there is the assumption that the activity will result in community betterment but the focus is clearly on the development of the individual and of the group-as-a-whole; the community benefits through the consequent better functioning of individuals and groups.

It can be seen that the boundary between casework and group work is not entirely clear. Group work is used to help individuals, and caseworkers are increasingly utilising the group as a helping medium such as in family casework and multiple interviews. Both are individually oriented and concerned with personal problems and personal development.

COMMUNITY ORGANISATION

The focus of community organisation is very different. Traditionally in the USA community organisation has meant the bringing together of organisations involved in social welfare so as to co-ordinate and develop their activities in order to meet community needs more adequately. Over time the meaning of the term has broadened to include a wide range of activities including that which is referred to as 'community work' in this country. One of the most elaborate attempts at a comprehensive definition – and certainly one of the most widely quoted – is that of Murray Ross:

> 'Community organisation . . . is . . . a process by which a community identifies its needs or objectives, orders (or ranks) these needs

or objectives, develops the confidence and will to work at these needs or objectives, finds the resources (internal and/or external) to deal with these needs or objectives, takes action in respect to them, and in so doing extends and develops co-operative and collaborative attitudes and practices in the community.'[8]

Insofar as 'community organisation' has been talked about in this country it has been in terms of the work of Councils of Social Service, Old People's Welfare Committees, Committees for the Physically Handicapped and similar organisations engaged in the co-ordination, promotion and development of the work of a number of bodies in a particular field at the local, regional or national levels.

This view comes from an analogy with the USA. But the development of social welfare in the USA has been along rather different lines. Until only just recently, most of the initiative for social welfare rested with the private sector. However, because so much of the responsibility for social services in the United Kingdom rests with the public sector the question arises as to whether activities similar to 'community organisation' can operate in the statutory social services.

SOCIAL ADMINISTRATION

The somewhat ill-defined and hybrid subject of social administration has always been an important element in the preparation of social workers in Britain. In the past, however, it was often focused on social legislation, on the structure and functions of services somewhat arbitrarily defined as 'social services' and on the development of national social policy. It has not been concerned with application or practice except possibly at higher levels of government.

In recent years there has been a growing interest in the processes of management and administration. Much of this interest, however, has been focused on the internal processes through which agencies are managed. Yet the external functions of the administrator, as they are described in Ross's definition of community organisation given above, would seem to be as important as internal management for the achievement of the agency's objectives. The relevance of these external functions to the administration of social services can best be appreciated in terms of their contribution to the resolution of community problems and to maintaining as well as changing the social service organisation.

This broader conception of administration is described clearly by Professor Donnison:

'Administration may be regarded as a set of procedures for linking those who control the resources for certain tasks . . . with those who use the goods or services produced from these resources (e.g. pupils, patients, tenants, customers). The Administrator has to maintain and develop collaboration between those who control or provide re-sources, those who perform the tasks that convert these resources into goods and services, and those who use the products or outcome of this work. If these three groups are not effectively and continuously linked the work cannot be done and the agency responsible for doing it will eventually go out of business.'[4]

Donnison describes the community organisation tasks of the agency administrator:

'Chief Officers are responsible for the agencies they direct but our studies show that some of the social services' most important tasks are performed by staff in several different agencies. . . . Fruitful development of the work often calls for the participation of many people outside the agency, and a willingness to subordinate the in-terests of the agency to those of the people to be served; otherwise the evolution of social policies may be frustrated or wastefully dis-torted.'[5]

He points out that the ability of social workers is 'to bring organisations other than their own to the aid of their clients, and to modify and develop the services within which they operate is no longer a peripheral concern but a central feature of their professional equipment'.[6]

COMMUNITY DEVELOPMENT

Another source of knowledge and experience for community work is 'community development' which derives from work in less-developed countries. Before the Second World War the development of colonial territories tended to be determined by the commercial and industrial interests of the imperial power. This led to economically large-scale but socially narrow development of mineral resources and agricultural products in mines and plantations, development which was heavily dependent upon foreign capital and expertise. After the war, with the pervading atmosphere of reconstruction and development, and with the emergence of militant nationalisms which led to the eventual political independence of the countries concerned, the attention of the govern-ments of these countries was increasingly concentrated on the problem of nation-wide social and economic development. The common aim was to accelerate the pace of development and to increase the amenities, skills and wealth of the people to match the rapid advance towards poli-tical independence and the rising level of social and economic expecta-tions. Community development emerged as a method to support national development and was defined by the Colonial Office in 1947 as 'a movement designed to promote better living for the whole community with the active participation and, *if possible,* on the initiative of the community, *but if this initiative is not forthcoming spontaneously, by the use of techniques for arousing and stimulating it'.*[7] With independence, many of the new governments in turn embraced community development as a means of nation building and of bringing about social and economic development.

The United Nations state that:

'The term "community development" has come into international usage to connote the process by which the efforts of the people themselves are united with those of governmental authorities to improve the economic, social and cultural conditions of communities, to integrate these communities into the life of the nation and to enable them to contribute fully to national progress.

'The complex of processes is thus made up of two essential elements: the participation of the people themselves in efforts to improve their level of living with as much reliance as possible on their own initiative, and the provision of technical and other services in ways which encourage initiative, self-help and mutual help and make them more effective. It is expressed in a variety of programmes designed to achieve a wide variety of specific improvements.'[8]

The two elements to which the definition refers, however, conceal a certain contradiction. Overseas community development emphasises participation, initiative and self-help by local communities but is usually sponsored by national governments as part of a national plan. While from one side it can be seen as the encouragement of local initiative and local decision making, from the other it is a means of implementing and expediting national policies at the local level and is a substitute for, or the beginning of, local government.

This objective distinguished overseas community development from community development in this country where the term was initially appropriated for work at the neighbourhood level with a primary emphasis on the autonomy and self-direction of the groups involved. It was seen as a process whereby community groups were assisted to clarify and articulate their needs and objectives and to take collective action in respect of them. It emphasised the involvement of the people themselves in determining and meeting their own needs. Early examples would include the Association of London Housing Estates[9] and the North Kensington Family Project.[10] More recently, central and local government have established community development projects which again broadens the conception.

Very often the emphasis in community development work is primarily educational. Dr Batten, one of the foremost advocates of community development, sees it primarily as an educational process aiming at personal growth towards self-direction and responsibility. Improvement in material conditions follows from changes in people and in their attitudes towards each other, rather than vice versa.[11]

COMMUNITY WORK

From this perspective, community development comes very close to group work as described earlier. In fact one might see the activities discussed hitherto as a continuum consisting of casework/group work/ community development/community organisation/social administration. While no clear-cut distinction is possible or desirable, the primary emphasis on the casework/group work end of the continuum is on individual and group development while on the other side it is on collective action in relation to the environment or community. We shall, therefore, use the term 'community work' to cover the broad range of activity on the far end of the continuum which includes work with community groups, administration and social planning.

An important distinction among these activities can be made in terms of the 'client'. In casework and group work this is relatively clear. With community development the situation becomes more complicated, for the people involved are explicitly or implicitly representative of a wider group on whose behalf they are acting, and the action proposed may well affect a still wider group, some of whom in fact may be in opposition to the proposal. In community organisation and social administration the conception of a 'client' in the casework sense is similarly complicated. In considering the practice of community work, one continuing source of confusion lies in the name itself, 'community work', for this seems to imply that one works with 'the community' or even 'the whole community'. One definition of 'community' is: 'the smallest territorial group that can embrace all aspects of human life. . . . It is the smallest local group that can be and often is, a complete society.'[12] For most people in our kind of society, however, the smallest territorial group that embraces all aspects of life would be very large indeed and would have few of the characteristics associated with the idea of a local community.

The author of the definition, in fact, goes on to modify his conception very radically when he writes: 'The modern community cannot be understood in terms of itself alone. Each segment may be more closely linked with similar segments in other communities than with dissimilar segments in the same community.'[13] The term 'community' in the more traditional sense of a geographical locality, still has meaning in certain villages, small towns and long-established neighbourhoods and for certain categories of people, particularly the aged, the very young, mothers of young families, the disabled and the poor. But in many places the geographical community has only a weak existence, and membership in various communities-of-interest unrelated to geographical propinquity is much more significant. In considering 'the community', therefore, we must take account of many different groups, networks and communities-of-interest interconnected in various ways and to varying degrees and occupying varying and overlapping territories. Often they are more strongly related to similar groups, networks and communities-of-interest outside the area than to others within it.

The word 'community' in community work is generally descriptive, rather like the term 'social' in social work, and does not give any precise guidance as to the entity with which the worker is concerned. The community worker rarely works with the whole community in terms of population or total interests. The worker must, of course, understand the broader social situation within which he is working and relate his activities appropriately to it. He needs an understanding of community structure and processes. But what he is working with is not a whole community but a system of inter-related individuals, families, groups, organisations and interests. Nor is the system a static entity that exists in plain view. It is defined in terms of the problem, need or interest at issue, the tasks to be undertaken and the purposes to be achieved. Inevitably, therefore, it changes over time.

A somewhat illogical but nevertheless useful distinction can be made between three major areas of community work: first, service development or the community work of the direct-service agency; second, inter-organisational co-ordination and social planning; and third, work with community groups.

SERVICE DEVELOPMENT

In considering service development or the community work of the direct-service agency, the focus is on an agency that is responsible for providing services to meet some specified need or problem. The service is usually associated with a particular consumer or client group such as children, the aged, or the physically or mentally ill. In order to carry out its service responsibilities the agency must engage in activities that support and enhance its basic function. The interest here is in the community work aspects of the agency's activities rather than in the techniques of direct service to individuals and families.

It is necessary for an organisation to mobilise resources in order to maintain itself. It must obtain the personnel, funds and facilities necessary to sustain its operations. In a highly competitive world in which money and staff are most often in short supply, a service agency must run fast just to stay in the same place. It is important to distinguish between the mobilisation of these resources and those concerned with the subsequent management of them. Community work is concerned with the former set of activities – how an organisation obtains resources from the community and how it plans to use them. Once the resources are in hand, the organisation carries out important internal activities that put them to use, such as staff supervision, financial control and office routines. These can be seen as management activities, which are not our main concern.

In order to obtain resources, an organisation must develop relationships with other groups and organisations that can help or hinder the attainment of its objectives. Thinking in terms of a casework agency, other individuals or bodies will affect the number and type of clients a service receives. The hospital, the general practitioner, the school, the housing department, the police, clergy, neighbours and many others may be important in this respect. Preventive work will be highly dependent on this process. Other bodies will be able to give or withhold information that will be important to the effective operation of the service such as medical assessments, school records and work records. Above all, other individuals and bodies control resources required by the clients of the service (e.g. access to treatments, residential placements, jobs, money, housing, training, foster-homes, group experience and recreational facilities). Relationships have to be established at the field or individual client level, as well as on an *ad hoc*, piecemeal basis, in response to crisis. In view of their importance to the welfare of clients, linkages with other organisations need to be developed on a sustained and systematic basis.

Agreement needs to be reached on who deals with what. The function and field of operation of the service must be formally or tacitly sanctioned by others involved. Difficulties in this area consequent on the expansion of services and a changed conception of service led to the reorganisation of the personal social services.

Another aspect of the community work of the direct-service agency, and one which is implicit in the two already mentioned, is bringing about changes in the quality or quantity of the resources necessary to provide adequate services to clients. Clients have needs which may not be adequately met by existing resources, so that it is desirable to change the existing arrangements in some way or to establish new provisions. This is a process in which all services are engaged to some extent. But although all services are engaged in the process it is often seen as something of a distraction from the main tasks of the service and not fully acknowledged as part of the ongoing functions of the staff that requires time, training, personnel and facilities.

Finally, a closely related community-work activity of a service agency is that of ameliorating or removing adverse social conditions that may underlie or aggravate the problems of clients such as inadequate income, bad housing and generally poor environmental conditions. Increasingly, as the complexities and connections among social problems is understood, the service agency is drawn into efforts to enhance the social welfare of the community it serves. Since this frequently requires joint thinking and action with other bodies to establish new services or to modify existing social policies, it merges into the area of inter-organisational work.

One difficulty in considering the community work of the direct-service agency is that it is often not a separated activity but inextricably interwoven with the total work of the organisation. Responsibility for community work cannot be confined to a particular worker or workers within an organisation. It is a system of tasks distributed throughout the organisation. In both statutory and voluntary organisations it is evident that staff and other participants at many different levels may play a part in community work, including: committee members, particularly the chairman; the director or chief officer; senior administrative and professional staff; and those responsible for the direction of the field operation of the service such as area officers, section heads or supervisors. All of these, as well as the field staff, will be involved to a varying degree depending on the nature of the problems and the type of action required. At any one level, more than one person may be carrying part of the responsibility. In some cases, specific staff members may have special responsibility for the community work of the organisation.

SOCIAL PLANNING

A second major area of community work is inter-organisation co-ordination and joint planning. Co-ordination clearly involves co-operation but goes beyond it. Co-ordination involves bringing parts into proper relation and this implies more deliberate and systematic attempts to link and order the parties to the co-operation and to develop agreed-upon policies and procedures between organisations.

Planning adds a further dimension to the discussion. Planning refers to a relatively systematic method of solving problems and achieving objectives. It is an activity concerned with proposals for the future, with the evaluation of alternative proposals, and with methods by which these proposals might be achieved. In this sense planning has been described as going through a job beforehand in one's imagination.

The need for co-ordination and joint planning between organisations springs from an inescapable dilemma. On the one hand there is the increasing realisation of the indivisibility of human need and human problems, whether at the level of the individual or the society. On the other hand everything cannot be done at the same time or by one organisation. The more comprehensive the organisation becomes, the more likely it will have to be broken down into various sub-parts and thus, problems of co-ordination recur. Tasks have to be broken down into appropriate elements and this division of labour is not only a practical necessity but has many benefits in terms of concentration of effort, specialisation and the development of expertise.

But however appropriate the breakdown of the total task into its various components and however carefully patterned the relations between these parts, problems of co-ordination will remain. These problems are rendered even more difficult by the changing nature of social needs and provisions. Moreover the problems relate not only to types of activity and clientele but also to the geographical area of operation of organisations and to the relations between different levels of organisations such as central government and local authority or national association and local branch.

The main distinguishing feature of inter-organisational co-ordination and planning is that it attempts to bring together the activities of independent or relatively independent organisations or sub-units of organisations. From this objective flow many of the characteristic problems of inter-organisational work.

If a co-ordinating body moves beyond servicing and supporting the existing situation to trying to bring about more substantial changes in social arrangements it must address the problems of changing the powers, responsibilities, prestige and resources of existing organisations. Not unnaturally, organisations tend to be cautious and wary about change. The more important the problem and the more radical the change proposed, the more likelihood that the organisation will resist the change. In an effort to get agreement and joint action, limitations and provisos and compromises may have to be accepted so that what starts out as a far-reaching proposal for change may end as a minimal adjustment of the existing position. In the long run, the action proposed may benefit everyone. In the short run, however, some will almost certainly benefit at the expense of others. In a situation of scarce resources, meeting one particular need will mean that some other specific interest will be relatively worse off.

What means are available for overcoming the obstacles to co-ordination? One approach is the *improvement of communication*. Efforts are aimed at opening up or improving channels of communication, making more information available, gathering facts about the matter at issue, interpreting people and organisations to each other, stimulating increased personal contact among the people involved, bringing people together to talk over problems, joint study of problems, development of joint activity on non-controversial matters, and so on.

The major assumption in these approaches is that problems of co-ordination come from lack of understanding of the matters at issue or the different parties' lack of understanding of each other. When this is the case these measures might well be effective. When there is a real conflict of interest, however, they are less likely to succeed and we must presumably accept that real differences of view do occur and that not all difficulties are due to misunderstandings or ignorance.

Another approach is to try and establish greater prominence for shared goals or superordinate goals. At a high level of generality this is fairly easy because most of the organisations with which we are concerned subscribe to the idea of 'improving human welfare'. But these very general objectives are capable of many interpretations. If differences between organisations are to be overcome, more specific and more compelling objectives need to be developed. A dramatic illustration of the process is provided from time to time by an outside event, a crisis affecting all the organisations involved.

A third approach is through the more systematic and ingenious development of exchanges between organisations. In order to achieve their own objectives, organisations need a variety of resources that are controlled by other bodies. The other bodies in turn will require various resources to achieve their objectives. If these needs can directly or indirectly be brought into some kind of relation with each other a pragmatic basis might be provided for co-ordination and joint planning short of any specific ideological commitment.

A fourth approach is through increasing the influence of the co-ordinating body. This is a chicken and egg problem, for organisations are unlikely to set out deliberately to create a body that has too much control over them. Nevertheless, co-ordinating bodies are able to increase their influence. One way is by developing special knowledge and experience. Another way is by developing functions that are, or become, important for the constituent bodies. The co-ordinating body becomes recognised as the organisation to represent or negotiate on behalf of its members. The co-ordinating body may be able to obtain resources of its own that can be used as an incentive in relation to the constituent bodies. If the co-ordinating body is able to appoint its own staff they may be able, through skill and commitment, to achieve a great deal with little in the way of power or formal authority.

There remain limits, however, to what can be achieved by inter-organisational co-ordination and planning. Eventually this activity must rely on some degree of consensus or potential consensus among those involved. When this does not exist or cannot be achieved, other methods have to be adopted if change is to be brought about.

The attempt to reach agreement may, at least temporarily, be abandoned and more overt pressure of various kinds brought to bear on the organisations concerned. Alternatively, efforts may be directed not so much at the organisations involved but at some higher authority that can make decisions about their activities. For example, problems of co-ordination of the personal social services have not proved solvable at the local level so that central government intervention has been necessary.

WORK WITH COMMUNITY GROUPS

In work with community groups the worker operates in direct, face-to-face interaction with users of services, with residents in a neighbourhood, or with others sharing a problem, interest or aspiration and with other people who provide services or make decisions affecting whatever is at stake. Such workers may be employed by either voluntary or statutory organisations to encourage community development in its broadest sense or to promote some quite specific purpose.

Community participation and neighbourhood organisation activities service the following purposes:

(1) Community involvement as a means of getting services to people who need them: this may involve the dissemination of information about services and community resources, increasing understanding and acceptance of services, contacting potential users and people in touch with those needing help and, thus, the development of preventive work.

(2) Community involvement as a means of feedback from the community and from the people being helped: this includes activities aimed at ensuring that services are appropriate and responsive to changing community needs and aspirations.

(3) Community involvement as a means of stimulating an increased sense of responsibility by the community for services and for people in need.

(4) Community involvement as a means of encouraging self-help and mutual aid: sometimes this objective assumes that social services are an unfortunate necessity and the aim is to achieve a situation where they are no longer necessary.

(5) Community involvement for the social and psychological benefits to be derived from participation: with this approach the achievement of concrete objectives is perceived as secondary to personal and group development and the strengthening of collaborative attitudes and community problem-solving capacity.

(6) Community involvement as a means of enabling people to take collective social action on matters of importance to them: this objective

may embrace a wide range of activity ranging from more conventional methods using the normal channels, negotiation and pressure, through to protest activities such as picketing, marches, demonstrations, sit-ins and strikes.

In practice, the purposes and activities outlined may be intermingled. But there are certain tensions between them. For example, emphasis on the value of participation may militate against effective administrative action and vice versa. Concern with the provision of individual services or mutual aid activities may work against social protest.

PROBLEMS AND ISSUES

Community work with the socially deprived is a slow process and makes heavy demands on staff and other resources. Conversely, groups of this type may be less effective in terms of participation and action. Under these circumstances should the organisers give priority to participation or to the achievement of concrete results? In point of fact, the tendency is for the more motivated, the more able, the more upwardly-aspiring people to participate in organisational life and to take positions of leadership. Faced with the necessity of attaining some tangible outcome, whether in the mounting of a demonstration or the arranging of a summer playscheme, the organisers will be under some pressure to rely on the more able and willing. The 'hard-to-reach' will need far more help and encouragement to continue participation.

Another issue arises from the relationship of neighbourhood groups to the agencies that assist or sponsor them and which may even have organised them in the first place. Without the assistance of skilled workers, neighbourhood groups in deprived areas have great difficulty in sustaining themselves. On the other hand, the acceptance of such help carries with it a measure of direction and control over the affairs of the local group – at the very least to the extent of making it awkward for the group to act in open conflict with the policies of the agency that employs the worker. It is, of course, in relation to more controversial issues that the strains develop.

This dilemma may arise when a statutory body encourages organisation of people in a neighbourhood. Once organised, the group may raise difficult questions and generate pressures against the very department that helped the group get on its feet or against another department of the same authority. This dilemma, however, is not limited to statutory agencies. It occurs in relation to any type of sponsoring organisation, however non-establishment, when issues arise affecting its sources of funds or other aspects of its responsibilities or activities, its values, policies, and its accepted ways of working.

This leads to a basic question concerning the possible effectiveness of neighbourhood organisation in achieving change. What can activity at this level accomplish and what is beyond its reach? Participation may overcome feelings of apathy, hopelessness and alienation. Self-help and mutual aid activities can be developed to the extent that those involved have the necessary resources. Neighbourhood action may be able to deal with problems of a local nature or those that can be resolved by local decisions. Thus, for example, action at this level can be successful in dealing with conditions in a particular school, certain practices of various local services, the conditions of housing or the behaviour of landlords.

It becomes increasingly difficult, however, for action that is taken only at the neighbourhood level to have an impact on the general issues that affect many neighbourhoods or whole cities and about which decisions are made by policy makers far beyond the confines of a neighbourhood. The major problems facing deprived areas – unemployment, housing, income-maintenance, health services and education – involve the reallocation of national resources; the kinds of decisions that are entailed in changes of this scope cannot be made at the local level.

Currently, in the personal social services, a major issue is the relationship between community action and the provision of services. These two types of activity, however, are not alternatives; they are different orders of intervention, addressed to different problems and with different immediate objectives in mind.

There are clearly many advantages in combining the two approaches. Community action and social service have in common the ultimate objectives of enabling people to cope with their life situations more effectively and of developing improved provision. Insofar as the approaches differ, each might be seen as a necessary support for the other. Without such support, community action might ignore the immediate needs of individuals in the interest of the collective cause, while personal social services might ignore the importance of such conditions and attempt to deal with community problems as though they were individual problems.

Nevertheless there are tensions between these approaches. The most important of these relate to the position of the agency in relation to other agencies and the community-in-general. Community action may identify the agency in such a way that while some clients may be attracted, others who are equally needy may be repelled. Community action may antagonise other organisations so that resources and services cease to be available to the agency's clients. Community action may so antagonise powerful forces in the wider community that the agency's entire operation is threatened.

This description of potential problems may give an unbalanced impression. With a wide range of constructive activities, insuperable difficulties are not likely to occur. The real problems arise when community action becomes actively involved in conflict over matters that are markedly controversial in the wider society upon which the agency and the worker are dependent for their support.

Beyond a certain point the worker's role moves, at least in the eyes of the wider community, from being primarily professional to being primarily political and beyond the terms of reference of the service. There is no absolute criterion for determining this point. It would seem to depend partly on the nature and level of the issues at stake and the remedies advocated, partly on the actual activity involved, partly on its relation to normal political activity and above all on the attitudes and policies of those who control the resources upon which the service is dependent.

The limits of the role of the worker and of the function of the service in community action are determined by the interactions among these factors, as well as by variations in place and time. Nor are workers necessarily passive in this situation. They can contribute to the definition of their role and it is part of their professional task and responsibility to the people and groups they service to assess the situation correctly and to maximise the possibilities for effective action. As yet, however, the conventions and rules have still to be established and generally accepted.

NOTES AND REFERENCES FOR CHAPTER 10

1 *Report of the Working Party on Social Workers in the Local Authority Health and Welfare Services*, para. 638, pp. 182-3
2 Harleigh B. Trecker, *Social Group Work: Principles and Practices* (New York: Associated Press, 1955), p. 5.
3 Murray Ross, *Community Organisation. Theory, Principle and Practice* (New York: Harper & Row, 1967), p. 39.
4 Donnison *et al.*, *Social Policy & Administration*, p. 36.
5 ibid., p. 248.
6 ibid., pp. 12-13.
7 Colonial Office, *Social Development in the British Colonial Territories* (London: HMSO, 1954). Report of the Ashridge Conference on Social Development, 3-12 August 1954.
8 UN, *European Seminar on Community Development and Social Welfare in Urban Areas* (Geneva: 1959), p. 1.
9 George Goetschius, *Working with Community Groups* (London: Routledge & Kegan Paul, 1969).
10 Roger Mitton and Elizabeth Morrison, *A Community Project in Notting Dale* (London: Allen Lane, 1972).
11 T. R. Batten with Madge Batten, *A Non-Directive Approach in Group and Community Work* (London: Oxford University Press, 1967).
12 Kingsley Davis, *Human Society* (New York: Macmillan, 1961), p. 312.
13 ibid., p. 315.

Chapter 11

COMMUNITY WORK AND SOCIAL WORK IN THE UNITED KINGDOM

Catherine Briscoe

The development of community work in Britain and the United States has been fashioned by influences such as sociological research, adult education, planning for social welfare services, community development in rural and traditional societies and the activities of radical reform and pressure groups.[1] However, in the United States the social work profession considers community work to be one of its methods, and most community work practitioners view themselves as being part of the profession of social work. They belong to the National Association of Social Workers and the current focus of concern in the profession is 'how social work through its community organisation arm will relate itself to broader social needs and pressures'.[2]

In Britain, community workers are considerably less clear about their professional identification, and they come from different backgrounds and work in a variety of settings. Some practitioners have social work training, but many have entered the field with sociology or political science degrees, with training in youth and community work, from housing and planning programmes, or with no educational or experimental preparation. They are employed in local authority departments responsible for housing, education, planning and social services, as well as in probation services, voluntary organisations and churches. The national government, too, has sponsored various community work activities.

The Association of Community Workers is organised independently of the British Association of Social Workers and explicitly recruits members on the basis of their interest and work in the field rather than on the basis of qualification. Many community work practitioners 'do not see social work as their reference point'. This is perceived 'not as an issue of principle, but because they see it as essential for community work to develop its own identity and its own methods of working independent of social work traditions and preoccupations'.[3]

However, despite separatist claims, social work's interest in community work has been increasing. Many social work agencies are employing community workers and/or encouraging their staff to use community work approaches. Courses of social work training are including information on community work and/or providing community work field experiences. This trend was given considerable impetus by the recommendations of the Seebohm Committee[4] to encourage social services departments to establish 'community oriented' family services. Local authority social services departments are now among the biggest employers of community workers in Britain; and other statutory and voluntary social work agencies are also employing community workers.

DEFINITION OF COMMUNITY WORK

Community work is a method that focuses on the ways in which peoples' physical and organisational environment furthers or hinders their wellbeing, and thereby promotes the interaction of individuals and groups living in the same community. The objective of community work is to enhance the capacity of communities to promote social functioning by strengthening resources, services and opportunities to meet various life tasks, alleviate distress and realise aspirations and values.[5]

The areas of intervention with which community workers are concerned vary. Some community workers are employed in small geographic localities such as housing estates or housing redevelopment neighbourhoods. Others work in wider geographical areas, such as the service area of a team in a social services department. And others work in large catchment areas with groups such as the elderly and ex-offenders. The communality of such groups arises from their common interests rather than from geographical closeness.

TYPES OF COMMUNITY WORK

The approaches that community workers and their employing agencies may use have been described and categorised by different writers. David Jones, in 'Community work in the United Kingdom' (Chapter 10), describes three kinds of community work in some detail:

(1) *service development* (or the community work of the direct-service agency) which focuses on the necessity for agencies both to understand the needs of the community and to develop support within the community to gain and maintain resources for the delivery of services;

(2) *inter-organisational co-ordination and planning* which is concerned with bringing agencies, departments and groups together to co-ordinate existing services and to plan jointly new resources and services;

(3) *work with community groups* where the worker concentrates on the development of groups in the neighbourhood or among specific populations to define their own needs and plan how to meet those needs.

The third of these approaches is the most widely discussed type of community work in Britain at the moment. However, the other two are practised, most notably in councils of social service and in statutory and voluntary agencies. It is our thesis that these different types of community work are complementary and should each contribute to the effectiveness of the others. But it should be recognised that there is a difference of focus between them. Service development and inter-organisational work and planning are essentially concerned with the *planning, organisation and delivery of services;*[9] that is, they concentrate on improving and developing agency output to client groups, both to improve existing services and to provide new services to enhance the quality of life.

Work with community groups is more concerned with direct intervention with community residents. It rests on the notion that problems exist within a particular locality that arise from the quality of interaction among residents and between residents and service providers. Further, this form of community work assumes that the locality can define its needs and interests, and that residents together with service providers and resources holders can respond to that definition.

Each of these two foci of community work (the planning, organisation and delivery of service and the work with community groups) is relevant and important to social work. The change objectives of community work range from information sharing to creating pressure for changes in legislation and policies affecting service-delivery systems.

Community-oriented community work and service-delivery-oriented community work are interdependent. The aims of community groups can be achieved only with the active co-operation and response of service providers and resource holders. This co-operation is most likely to be forthcoming if there is information sharing and co-ordination with service providers. Service-delivery goals can be met only through the active participation and involvement of community residents and service consumers. Neither set of objectives can be pursued in isolation from the other. In pursuing their goals, both the community and the service organisation should appreciate their interdependence.

In Table 1 examples of the range of tasks in both forms of community work are shown, beginning with tasks of changing people and developing their capacities to use available services and resources, and ending with tasks that demand fundamental change in the organisation and distribution of services and resources.

Many social workers and social agency management staff will recognise, in the list of the service-delivery oriented tasks, work that they already carry out with varying degrees of emphasis. We identify them as community work tasks and point out their use to the social work agency in order to emphasise their importance in the social work agency. Community work knowledge and skill, insofar as it is presently developed, provides the practice base for these tasks. Community-oriented tasks are less accepted as an integral part of practice by social workers and administrative staff. The value of this form of practice to the agency is less well recognised and frequently the subject of controversy. These activities can be viewed as a means of enabling people to articulate and find ways to meet their own needs.

Table 1   Community Work Tasks

Service-Delivery Oriented	*Community Oriented*
(1) *Developing an information flow* collecting information from the community on needs and feeding it into the agency giving out information on existing needs, services and resources	(1) *Improving access to services and resources for community residents* setting up information centres putting information into the hands of community residents providing information about services
(2) *Developing and improving service resources* drawing in volunteers, other professionals, community groups and financial resources to aid service delivery helping agency staff to use resources and contacts	(2) *Developing community support and service linkages and resources* recruiting volunteers setting up care schemes setting up visiting schemes self-help groups
(3) *Developing and improving services* co-ordinating and planning with service providers getting feedback from the community examining access to provision and flexibility of response to the needs of special groups sharing feedback and planning with agency staff	(3) *Participation of community residents in service planning* representation in co-ordination groups collection and provision of information on needs and effects of service

Table 1 (*continued*)

Service-Delivery Oriented	Community Oriented
(4) *Development of new services, facilities and resources for client groups* consultation with groups co-ordination with other services advocacy and interpretation to resource holders and decision makers planning, development, and governing new resources with client groups and agency staff	(4) *Gaining new resources and facilities for the community* forming issue-oriented groups documenting needs and finding ways of meeting them formation of pressure groups and support groups locating and negotiating for resources
(5) *Provision for special needs of a specific client group* consultation with groups interpretation and advocacy to resource holders, decision makers and the public	(5) *Changing relative status of groups* political and technical education public relations finding resources and backing
(6) *Attempt to change policy provisions and legislation* collection of information presentation of information with proposals advocacy and publicity through agency system, developing staff support public relations	(6) *Attempt to change policy provisions or legislation* formation of issue and pressure groups collection and presentation of information use of political tactics publicity and campaigning

The list does not constitute a comprehensive catalogue of either service-delivery-oriented or community-oriented community work tasks. They are examples drawn from the practice of a number of community workers and social workers. Nor are the tasks listed as distinct and separate as they appear. In either form of community work, task activities fluctuate and develop from one focus to another. In community-oriented activities a group that is formed for self-help and community support may become involved in hunting for resources and move into negotiating with resource holders. An example would be a mothers' group that decides to organise a playgroup and needs money and space to do so.[7] Similarly, in service-delivery-oriented activities, volunteers who are recruited to help individual clients may become involved in a campaign for new services to help particular client groups or for changes in policy provisions and legislation to remedy visible deficiencies in existing provisions. For example, volunteers who work with the elderly have become involved in campaigns for higher pension rates.

The difference between the two emphases described here are also more blurred in practice than Table 1 suggests. Community work practitioners frequently find themselves supporting community groups of all kinds and at the same time attempting to recruit volunteers or develop co-ordinating patterns among a range of service providers. The theoretical division is useful to demonstrate the divergence of objective and perspective involved in the two kinds of tasks. The worker employed by an agency and working with a community often finds himself caught in a conflict of priorities between the two forms of work and it is useful to be able to clarify for the agency, for the community and for himself, the priorities he gives to either of the two perspectives.

Agencies and community groups frequently have very different perceptions of priorities. Feedback and exchange with service agencies and the development of caring schemes and volunteer resources may be given low priority by area residents. On the other hand, agencies may feel threatened rather than helped in their service-delivery tasks by the priorities of community groups which may bring extra demands on their resources, criticism of their procedures and angry reactions from other agencies or departments that are also exposed to such demands and criticisms. Agencies that employ community work specialists or that encourage social workers to relate closely to the community may see service-delivery-oriented community work as most useful and most relevant to their own goals and functions. However, the value of community work lies only partly in the improved services that may result and in the interactions between community people and the agency. From the perspective of community residents, the most positive benefits may lie

(a) in the learning that takes place in interaction with others, and in participation in decision making; and
(b) in the strengthened ability of groups to cope with the complex forces that affect their daily lives.

While a social work agency may not enjoy the criticisms and demands for resources brought to it as a result of work with community groups, the increased knowledge of problems that accrues from these efforts puts the agency in a better position to understand and support the efforts of community groups to change social conditions and to influence resource holders.

Many community workers may see service-delivery-oriented activities as irrelevant to the needs of the community. They frequently describe them as 'exploiting' the community or 'using community residents to do the job of the social work agency'. They do not appreciate community members' needs for social support from each other, the interest of community members in helping each other, nor the need for social services to receive information, feedback and help from the community so that they can provide an accessible, relevant and caring service.

Both foci of community work appear important and appropriate for social work agencies. But it is crucial for an agency and its staff to be clear about, and agreed upon, the priorities given to either emphasis.

COMMUNITY WORK KNOWLEDGE AND SKILLS

Community work activities require knowledge and skills that are common to both social work and community work. The CCETSW Paper[*] on training for community work points out that there are also knowledge and skills specific to community work. Here we shall mention briefly some areas of knowledge and skill that are essential for community work:

(1) The community worker must be able to work with the client-system, with his own agency and with other service providers in a manner that wins interest and involvement. The community worker is dependent on a wide range of interests and commitment from others to achieve change of any sort. Maintaining a clear view of goals while prevailing on others to commit time and energy to work towards agreed-upon goals requires self-knowledge, understanding of the motivations of others and flexibility in forming working relationships.

The community worker must locate, define and reach out to client systems and to action systems and persuade them that he has something to offer. He has to awaken consciousness of problems and build the belief that something can be done about them.

(2) To build constituencies through planned interactions with a variety of people, the community worker must be skilled in understanding the perspectives and concerns of individual persons as well as in communicating a community-wide problem analysis.

(3) The community worker must know how to assess the community in which he works in terms of its problems, issues and resources. This includes knowing where to get information and being able to evaluate it in order to identify problems and resources related to localities and population groups.

(4) To help groups formulate a programme to effect change, the community worker needs to know how to acquire and communicate information about structures of decision making and influence re-

lated to the problem, and about alternative solutions. He must be able to see a problem in its wider context (such as how it affects the interests of other groups and organisations), to understand the relevance of the wider context to the group's interests and to communicate his understanding to the group. This requires knowledge about political and organisational structures and about strategies for dealing with them.

(5) The community worker must be able to recognise when groups and individuals can carry tasks themselves and when they need his help. Groups must be allowed to move at their own speed and to assume responsibilities as they are ready.

(6) Communication skills are particularly important for the community worker, who must be able to: write and help others write reports that are easily read, hold the attention and prove their points; find ways of helping groups gain access to and use the media; and persuade individuals and groups to consider ideas that may be contrary to their own.

(7) As the community worker is involved with groups of residents, with service providers and with decision makers, he must find ways of helping them to relate to one another. Being able to discuss issues from different angles with different groups and to explain and interpret one group to another without usurping the right of any one group to talk and negotiate directly with the other is a fundamental community work skill.

CHOICES IN COMMUNITY WORK INTERVENTION

Community workers must make choices as to the focus of their practice. No community worker can hope to work with all individuals, families and groups in a community or population group. A community worker must choose, firstly, the source of stress upon which he will concentrate; secondly, the network of individuals and groups in the population with which he will work; and, lastly, the particular role behaviour he will adopt in working with these issues and networks. These choices are guided by three factors. First, there are *the objectives of the employing agency* which will provide varying degrees of clarity of focus. For example, the Age Concern organisation indicates clearly that workers should focus on stress in the elderly arising from ageing and from their treatment by society. Social services departments, on the other hand, allow for a wide range of options in the choice of issues and networks.

Although some agencies, particularly statutory ones, are beginning to advocate a 'low profile' stance for a community worker, few agencies define the actual manner in which the community worker should pursue his chosen objectives. Generally speaking, the worker can determine for

himself from the agency's policies and procedures, and from his knowledge of the sanctions and sponsorship under which the agency operates,
what kind of role behaviour will be most effective in that setting.

Second, *the character and structure of the community* determines, in
part, about what, with whom, and how, the worker will proceed. The
worker undertakes study and assessment of the community to learn
about sources of stress, who is affected by them and who is interested
in doing something about them. Existing pressure groups and organisations and potential allies are located through this process.

Third, these choices are affected by the *community worker's political
and philosophical stance* and by his value assumptions.

These last influences on choice of focus are controversial and, in
agencies where community workers have been left to define their own
job description, this has created misunderstanding. There is also considerable disagreement about this among community work practitioners
themselves. While it is not possible to discuss all elements of value conflict in community work in this space, it will be useful to describe some
of the philosophical assumptions that create conflict.

VALUES IN COMMUNITY WORK

The value assumptions in community work that affect practitioners'
choices arise from the objectives of community work. The Gulbenkian
Group outlined three value assumptions that they felt would be widely
agreed upon by community workers. First, they stated that 'people
matter and that policies, administrative systems and organisational practices should be judged by their effect on people'. Second, 'people acting
together develop their capacities as human beings. A society should give
maximum opportunity for the active participation of people in every
aspect of the environment, social, economic and political.' The third
assumption relates to the need for sharing and redistribution of power
in any society or community that is genuinely concerned about social
equality and social justice.[9]

Although there may be a high degree of consensus between community workers and sponsoring agencies on these assumptions, basic
disagreements occur when it comes to identifying the blocks that prevent
people from participating in the control of their environment. In the
view of some, the blocks lie in the incapacities of individuals to use and
advance themselves within the existing social and political system. The
historical influences of puritanism in our culture support the belief that
those who wish to better themselves can do so provided they have no
obvious mental or physical handicaps to prevent it. Others perceive the
blocks to lie in the structure of a society that discriminates against
deprived groups, keeping the poor in poverty. How service providers

and fieldworkers perceive these blocks affects their perspectives about the causes of social problem.

Problem definitions range along a continuum from an individual-incapacity orientation to a structural-deficiency orientation as illustrated below:

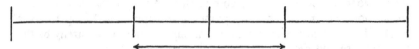

Problems exist because of the incapacities of individuals

Problems exist because of a combination of individual incapacities and structural insufficiencies

Problems exist because of the structural deficiencies of society

Change objectives related to these perspectives constitute a similar continuum ranging from changing individuals in order to help them cope better with their situation to changing the structure of society to make it more relevant to the needs of its members. Most community workers perceive problems to be rooted to some extent in the capacity of people to use existing resources and services. But they place greater stress on the availability of resources, and on policies and programmes for their distribution. Although most community workers would place themselves towards the structural end of this continuum, there are many variations in the emphases taken by different community workers. Differences in the emphasis given to one or another of these perspectives lead to conflicting views about the issues upon which community work should focus. For example, one practitioner might believe that problems of loneliness and isolation among community residents should have first priority, while another worker, perhaps in the same agency, might focus upon issues of housing policy and provision.

Similarly, one worker might concentrate on work with neighbourhood groups in self-help projects with the educational process of the work as his primary focus. Another worker in the same agency might give less emphasis to what the group members are learning and more emphasis to helping the group achieve a change in the institutional forces affecting their lives.

The worker's stance may also incline him either to work most closely with the people who are affected by the deficiencies in society or to work with the political decision makers who are in a position to bring about change.

DILEMMAS AND ISSUES IN COMMUNITY WORK

Because of misunderstanding about community work and social work objectives and activities, social workers and community work practitioners are often suspicious of one another. Frequently community workers view social work as a device to support the *status quo* by help-ing the individual adapt to an unjust social structure. Some social workers believe that community workers neglect the needs of individuals. There is little understanding of the complementary role of each form of social work although, in fact, community workers refer individuals to social workers, and community groups give support and help to social work clients. Clients who use casework support may have strengths that they can use and develop in community work activities.

Frequently, social workers distrust the capacity of community groups to help others in the community and believe that their aid is a poor substitute for the skilled help of the caseworker. Community workers, conversely, suspect social workers of fostering dependency and of providing help that is less 'natural' than that of a friend or neigh-bour.

Greater understanding of each other's activities could be brought about by much more information sharing and interchange among wor-kers. But because they are so heavily involved in their own activities they seldom find time to discuss mutual concerns and to explore their respec-tive contributions to agency goals.

Conflicting political and philosophical beliefs about practice may cause difficulties. Community workers may be seen as too radical because they are primarily oriented to structural change. In fact, community workers and social workers share a range of philosophies that might place mem-bers of each group in a variety of positions on our previously described continuum of change orientation. In deciding on courses of action all workers should be influenced primarily by the needs of the client system and the client system's perception of the problem rather than by their own personal philosophies. The shared value base of community work and social work emphasises the right and the need of the client system to determine its own goals. While this is a value that both social workers and community workers may sometimes violate in practice, there is nothing inherent in the value base of either form of practice that denies this value.

A final dilemma in community work practice relates to the conflict that may arise between a community group and the worker's agency. Where such conflict occurs, the community worker employed by the service-giving network is likely to be caught between the community and the network. His role is to try and build bridges across the gap and to help the community gain some response from the service network. An employing agency needs to recognise that if the community worker's activities have value, his ties to the community must be supported even when they create problems and discomfort for the agency. The com-munity worker must recognise also his responsibility to meet the needs of the service network for information and feedback in order to plan more flexible and relevant responses to community needs.

CONCLUSION

In spite of these problems, community work approaches are crucial to social work. They are a means of gaining understanding of the needs and resources in the community, developing strengths in the community to cope with sources of stress, developing services that are relevant to agency clients and articulating ideas for change that will reduce social problems.

The complexity of community work knowledge and skills requires that community workers have opportunities for training. The diversity and range of community work activities are indicative of the need to employ community workers at different levels in social work agencies. In addition, other social workers need knowledge and encouragement to use community resources and contacts developed by specialist community workers. While most social workers use community resources and perform some community work functions, it is important that these functions be made more explicit and that they become a central part of social work activity.

Above all, social work managers require a clear understanding of what community work can offer both to their agencies and to their clientele. They need to be able to define the priority tasks of community work in relation to their own agency. Once this is reasonably clear, job descriptions can be drawn up and staff appointed who are able to carry out these tasks. When given appropriate agency support and direction, community work can contribute to the improvement of the agency's service to its clientele and to the improvement of the life opportunities of the people the agency serves.

NOTES AND REFERENCES FOR CHAPTER 11

1 See: Arnold Gurin, 'Social planning and community organisation', p. 1324; Marjorie Mayo, *Community Development and Urban Deprivation* (London: National Council of Social Service, Bedford Square Press, 1974; Philip Bryers, 'Community work: current ideas and practice', *The Planner* (September/October 1973), pp. 354–6.
2 Arnold Gurin, 'Social planning and community organisation', p. 1333.
3 Central Council for Education and Training in Social Work, *The Teaching of Community Work*, Social Work Curriculum Study, CCETSW, Paper No. 3 (July 1974).
4 *Report of the Committee on Local Authority and Allied Personal Services.*
5 Pincus and Minahan, *Social Work Practice*, ch. 2.

6 Violet Sieder, 'The community organisation of the direct service agency', in Kramer and Specht (eds), *Readings in Community Organisation Practice*.
7 Mitton and Morrison, *Community Project in Notting Dale*.
8 CCETSW, *The Teaching of Community Work*, section 11, pp. 18 and 19.
9 Calouste Gulbenkian Foundation, *Community Work and Social Change*, ch. 2.

Chapter 12

RESIDENTIAL SOCIAL WORK

Chris Payne

INTRODUCTION

'People are both fascinated by and drawn towards their disowned bad objects and at one moment want to take them in and feel especially responsible for them and then at the next moment, equally without knowing why, find it vitally important to have them "out there", outside themselves in a place of safety. On the one hand, this splitting process goes on, the taking in of good objects, and the expulsion of bad ones; yet at the same time, there is also a pull towards the bad objects, which is often quite blind and unconscious.'[1]

We begin our discussion of residential work with Richard Balbernie's statement because it comprehends so accurately the complex relationships that pertain to different forms of institutional care in our society. Balbernie creates an awareness of the dilemmas of those at the interface, who have responsibilities for developing, administering and operating these social services. He implies that separation and integration are closely related human responses. This relationship is reflected in the ambivalence that is associated with many of the issues affecting residential practice. We become aware of this ambivalence in all discussions of the social policies that determine the shape, scope and purposes of residential provision, as well as the administrative structures through which these policies are implemented and the professional status of the people who manage residential units.

In this chapter, it is our intention to discuss the concept of integration as it pertains to this field of social service from several perspectives: first, we shall examine the relationship of residential care to the supportive and preventive social services and consider the organisation and administration of residential services. Then we shall discuss the development of residential work and the struggle of residential workers to find a professional identity. Throughout the discussion we will attempt to keep under consideration the needs of the residents for whom social integration is of vital importance. We hope to apprise readers of the conflicting views that are held in regard to this heterogeneous area of social services, and of the many problems that are encountered in developing positive and constructive approaches to residential care.

IS RESIDENTIAL CARE A PART OF COMMUNITY CARE?

Social policies of the past two or three decades have been directed to finding alternatives to residential care. Social policy has also been concerned with improving the standards of care of those for whom there are not alternatives to residential care. The main objective of current policy is to eliminate the Poor Law notion of residential care which sought to remove socially deprived and destitute people from the community to 'places of safety' that were distinguished by the size, shape and location of the buildings. In such places, the recipients were often considered to be beyond the pale of normal society. Current social policy supports the idea of 'community care' whereby residential care is seen as a social service to enable dependent people to remain in the community without fear of stigma, to retain their identity by maintaining links with members of their family and with friends and to achieve as much independence as possible within the limitations of their handicaps.

Residential Child Care

Many changes in residential care have taken place since the end of the Second World War. In child care they are manifest in family group homes and other small children's homes that complement the extensive use of boarding-out facilities and that reduce the need for 'cottage homes' and large barrack-like institutions. Extensive use is now made of facilities for observing and assessing children who require residential care in order to place them appropriately according to their needs.

In child care the 1969 Children's and Young Persons' Act is perhaps the most recent attempt to implement the philosophy of community care. It provides the framework for an integrated system of community homes for all children in need of care including juvenile offenders who, formerly, had been committed to approved schools. Under the 1969 Act the title of 'approved school' has been abolished. Many of these previously independent schools are now administered as community homes by local authorities. The intention of this reorganisation is to develop a comprehensive system of care by establishing residential and non-residential treatment programmes. The non-residential treatment programmes, usually called 'intermediate treatment', are intended to fill a preventive function by providing compensatory and remedial experiences for children who are under supervision. Existing resources, such as youth clubs and playgroups, are used flexibly and with discrimination to develop intermediate treatment. Specialist facilities are developed in some programmes; and some programmes provide for children to spend short periods away from home. The aim is to provide a network of services in each area so that children who are at risk or who have been in trouble with the law can be treated according to their particular needs.

The intense controversy over the implementation of the 1969 Act is a salutary reminder of the numerous difficulties that must be overcome before comprehensive services for young people can be established. Commonly, local communities express ambivalence towards proposals to treat deviant members within the community. Currently this ambivalence is reflected in many ways: widespread concern about the shortage of residential accommodation and special facilities for disturbed and disruptive youngsters; juvenile magistrates complaining of their loss of authority to detain recalcitrant young people in places of safety; social workers being castigated for their overly permissive approach of allowing young offenders to remain at home after Care Orders have been made; social workers finding it difficult to secure residential places. One result of a generally unsatisfactory situation is that there has been an increase in the number of juveniles remanded to prisons and committed to Borstal training since the passage of the 1969 Act. This clearly defeats the objectives of the Act.

Unfortunately, the 1969 Children's and Young Persons' Act increased the responsibilities of local authorities during a period when general reorganisation was taking place. Because of this, local authorities have not been able to develop comprehensive care systems. In particular the development of intermediate treatment programmes has been retarded as a result of reorganisation. Co-ordination of the services that would constitute an integrated system often fails because social services departments separate the administration of the residential services from community (i.e. fieldwork) services. Additional problems are created in some departments where the development of intermediate treatment programmes is made the responsibility of personnel who belong to neither of the main operational divisions. The regional planning committees which have the responsibility for monitoring and co-ordinating the development of the community homes system and programmes of intermediate treatment are criticised for being too removed from the local situation to function effectively.

Residential Facilities for Adult Offenders
There have been corresponding developments of alternatives to imprisonment for adult offenders. These include community service orders and a more flexible use of hostel provision. Some hostels have a preventive function while others provide for rehabilitation and after-care. Experiments are also taking place in the use of 'bail' hostels, which provide

accommodation for people, who would otherwise be remanded to prison while awaiting trial.

Residential Care for Adults

In areas of social service other than child care the overall design is similar. It is to have a network of services that provide supportive and preventive functions, with residential care considered as an integral part of the total provision. This conception is being applied in planning for care of the chronically sick and physically disabled, the mentally ill, the mentally handicapped, and in care of the elderly. Local authorities and voluntary organisations are providing services for these groups including permanent and semi-permanent accommodation for people who cannot live independently or with their families and who might be otherwise confined unnecessarily to long-stay hospital wards. Many elderly people are able to remain in their own homes because of improved domiciliary and day-care services. Modern homes have replaced many grim Poor Law institutions for elderly people who need continuous care and attention. In addition, some local authorities have opened homes to provide intensive care for frail and confused elderly people.

As in child care, the implementation of policies of community care in these areas is rarely smooth or consistent. Titmuss once described the concept of 'community care' as 'a new concept, a new idea, a more promising health and social hybrid'; but, he added, 'it has to grow in the soil we have'.[2] Titmuss deplored the policy of discharging patients from mental hospitals when there are not a sufficient number of qualified social workers to provide supportive community services. He maintained this would have the effect of maintaining an illusion of community care.

There is, still, inadequate development of residential services for many groups such as hostels for the mentally ill and the mentally handicapped, and accommodation for the single homeless. In these cases supply has failed to meet the need. In some cases the lack of development in both quantitative and qualitative terms is attributable to the inability of the different agencies concerned to act in concert. And in many instances it is attributable to the shortage of trained and qualified residential workers who have the ability to develop these services.

INTEGRATION OR SEGREGATION?

Geographical Isolation

Those concerned with the integration of the residential services face the problem of deciding how to make effective use of available resources. The residential establishments that actually deliver services to these client groups are often not able to exercise integrative and rehabilitative functions because of their geographical isolation. This is particularly true in the case of the former approved schools and some institutions for the physically and mentally handicapped. New methods and ways of utilising these resources have still to be discovered.

Geographical isolation is not always without merits. It is possible to develop projects with imagination and discernment that overcome this particular problem. As the account of one intermediate treatment[a] project has revealed, geographical isolation can enhance the therapeutic potential of the residential situation. In this case a remote area was chosen as the setting for a programme offering a *limited* period of residential living to provide groups of young people with opportunities to work *intensively* on their adjustment problems.

Separatist Policies

A second problem that confronts those who are attempting to develop an integrated approach in residential care is to decide the degree of specialisation that is desirable among residential care units. Since the Second World War many large multi-purpose institutions have been replaced by smaller units that are organised on the basis of the age, sex, type of handicap or problematic behaviour of the clients. Thus, in child care the range of establishments controlled by a social services department may include: a residential nursery for infants and toddlers; separate homes for school-age children; homes for adolescent girls; homes for adolescent boys; hostels for working girls; hostels for working boys; special units for emotionally disturbed children; community homes for delinquent and maladjusted boys; and community homes for delinquent and maladjusted girls. In the field of education, separate residential schools are provided for maladjusted, physically handicapped and educationally subnormal pupils. For adults there are separate residential homes for the chronically sick and physically disabled, hostels for the mentally ill and homes for the mentally handicapped. There are residential homes for the elderly and separate homes for the elderly frail and for the elderly confused.

This specialisation of services is attributable, in part, to the growing use of a medical model to define and meet needs; it is also due, in part, to the piecemeal development of the social services. These policies have some negative consequences. First, feelings of rejection and stigma tend to be reinforced when groups of people are segregated according to their handicap and type of disability. Their sense of alienation is thereby likely to increase. Similarly, when people are separated on the basis of different types of deviancy their conceptions of themselves as deviant are likely to be reinforced. A second disadvantage of a separatist policy is that it narrows the range of social characteristics of the resident's peer group and diminishes opportunities for development of social relationships that are necessary for individual growth.

The influence of the peer group on the attitudes and behaviour of young delinquents in residential care has been the subject of many empirical studies, notably those carried out by Polsky in the USA.⁴ Similar findings have been obtained from studies with other client groups in residential care. For example, from his study of special homes for the elderly confused, Meacher has concluded that feelings of isolation and confusion are intensified when groups of old people are isolated from others in residential situations.⁵ Thus, the tasks of rehabilitation may be made more difficult by creating specialist units.

Administrative Divisions

Another manifestation of the separation of residential services from other forms of social service can be found in their organisation and administration. Since the reorganisation of the local authority social services departments, most residential establishments have been administered as separate divisions of the departments. Some argue that this separation has far-reaching implications for the development of residential services and their integration with other forms of social service. Righton believes that these divisions are not dictated simply on the basis of efficiency and administrative expediency. Rather, he suggests, they are related fundamentally to the values placed on different social services.⁶ He says:

'If society in general and the social services in particular, set a high value on the family and a low one on any alternative form of socialisation (outside the public boarding schools) it is likely from the outset that family and non-family services will be separately administered and that the allocation of resources will be weighted in favour of the former at the expense of the latter. What is in principle likely is what happens in fact.'

Thus, Righton suggests, residential services are starved of resources and are not managed by people with relevant experience and appropriate professional qualifications. He observes:

'Each service normally has an assistant director at the head of it. But whereas the assistant director in charge of field work services is, usually, a qualified social worker with substantial experience of the work he directs, only rarely has his colleague (in residential care) spent a single day as a residential practitioner. And even more rarely does he hold a relevant professional qualification. Distinctions of a related kind can be found from top to bottom of the hierachy.'

This catalogue of relative deprivations, maintains Righton, guarantees the perpetuation of residential care as a 'Cinderella service'. He concludes:

'The widespread conviction that residential care is an inferior alternative to family-type living is bound, if the present situation remains unchanged, to become a self-fulfilling prophecy. The mechanism is depressingly simple; first, predict that residential experience will damage people; then starve your residential services of the very resources that could enable you to prove yourself wrong.'[7]

Attitudes to Residential Care

As an integral part of social services, residential care must be seen as the preferred treatment in appropriate circumstances. Decisions regarding assignment to services must be based on assessment of a client's need. In this view the different social services should be seen as complementing one another in the total scheme of things. However, in practice the value the community sets on different services varies considerably. Residential care appears to be valued considerably less than other forms of social service. As the community's emphasis on prevention has increased, residential care has come to be perceived as a residual service. It is rarely considered to be the preferred treatment, and it is used only as a last resort when all else fails. Frequently this is the view of social workers who, because of their professional ideology, are committed to preventing admission to residential care under almost any circumstances. Some social workers interpret the admission of a client to care as their own failure to utilise properly their preferred method of intervention.

This trend is reflected in the changing population of residential homes. Many children's homes tend to admit only the most difficult, disturbed and socially handicapped children for whom community-based approaches and foster care are not available. In admissions to homes for the elderly over the last few years, there has been an increase in average age on admission and degrees of infirmity and handicap. However, these changes have often gone unrecognised or, if recognised, they have the tacit approval of the community and the professions. Thus residential homes have had imposed on them a highly specialised role. However, they have not been given the resources, particularly in the form of trained and qualified staff, to perform these complex tasks. As the tasks of these institutions have become more complex it has become more difficult to maintain high standards of care. This has the effect of maintaining residential care as a residual service.

An intense lack of confidence in the growth-enhancing possibilities of residential living lies beneath many of the administrative and professional policies that support this pattern of starving residential care of resources. An abundance of psychological studies on separation and sociological studies of the 'total institution' have contributed substantially to the idea that residential child care must always be an inferior alternative to family care. Unfortunately, the general public, elected representatives, administrators and members of the professions who believe that residential experiences are damaging or bad rarely ask how alternatives to family living can be developed as a constructive and creative experience.

Wolins,[8] after examining residential child care practices in several countries, has concluded that group care is as effective as other kinds of care in assisting the emotional, social, moral and intellectual development of children, provided that certain conditions are fulfilled. He suggests that the following are the ingredients of a successful group care situation:

(1) A clear-cut system of values on which policies and practices are based.
(2) Staff with a sense of optimism and commitment towards the task generated by having well-defined goals;
(3) An element of predictability, for staff and children, based on attitudes that the present placement is the most constructive one in the circumstances.
(4) The integration of the setting into the community so that the aims of the setting are fully understood and given recognition by members of the community.
(5) The development of healthy peer-group influences so that adults and children work together on the basis of common values and expectations.
(6) Engagement of the children in socially constructive activities to give them a sense of competence and ownership, which assists the development of a sense of identity.

There is ample evidence to be concerned about the extent to which these conditions exist in residential practice in Great Britain, not only in respect of the care of children but for all client groups in need of residential care.[9]

The therapeutic and educational potential of residential care have been recognised and exploited for many years by a long line of distinguished practitioners engaged in the residential treatment of emotionally damaged children and mentally ill adults. 'Milieu therapy' (or 'planned environment therapy', the term commonly used in Great Britain) and 'therapeutic communities' make explicit use of the processes of daily living as part of a programme of planned intervention. However, these ideas are virtually unused in most residential settings. By and large, resources are devoted to the limited objectives of providing the basic necessities of life.

The neglect of the residential living situation is nowhere better illustrated than in Oswin's *The Empty Hours*.[10] Oswin contrasts the bleak living conditions endured by severely physically handicapped and mentally subnormal children in long-stay hospital wards to those in other settings. Their lives contrast with those of children in some residential schools managed by voluntary organisations where exhaustive efforts are made to involve the children in the processes of daily living. The situation described by Oswin is, in some degree, characteristic of the entire field. Another study, dealing with care of children, shows that leisure and recreational periods are rarely used to provide compensatory experiences for the socially and culturally disadvantaged children in residential care.[11]

Miller and Gwynne's[12] description of residential care for chronically sick and physically disabled adults follows a similar pattern. There is a sharp contrast in the practices of the units studied. In some units residents are encouraged to be self-dependent and to participate in the decision making of the home; in others they are treated like hospital patients. Residential homes for the elderly are also often organised in accordance with a 'hospital' model where residents have to succumb totally to the ministrations of the staff. Residents are, in consequence, maintained in states of helplessness and dependency because situations that do not fit into the model of the physically helpless patient who is sustained by the nurse and physician are ignored.

DEVELOPMENT OF RESIDENTIAL WORK

Several years ago Titmuss[13] remarked that 'We have invested too much spiritual capital in structural goals and buildings (in anatomy) and not enough in this matter of the roles, functions, and responsibilities of workers in the field of health and welfare'. How correct he was. And how little have his warnings been heeded in considering the development of residential work. At the present time, with about 395,000 people in residential care and 65,000 staff members caring for them, less than 4 per cent of the latter have any training for residential work at all.[14] When one considers the heterogeneity of this field of social service it is not surprising that most of the people responsible for the day-to-day care of residents have only a flimsy professional identity.

There are many reasons for the slow development of residential work as a professional undertaking. We have already discussed how society's view of residential care as 'residual' affects the quality of these services. In addition, common elements in residential work have been submerged in the proliferation of specialisations in post-war provision which has retarded development of unifying principles. As a result, large numbers of people working in residential care have no training at all, and those who do receive their basic training in a variety of disciplines such as teaching and nursing. Frequently the only qualifications of residential workers are their personal attributes. Accordingly there has been virtually no career structure in residential work and some categories of employment (e.g. care assistants in residential homes for the elderly) are classified as 'manual workers' with weekly rates of pay. Others (e.g. child care staff from assistant level upwards) are paid monthly. The same position may be designated by a variety of role descriptions in different establishments. For example, the same job in children's homes may be described as 'warden', 'matron', 'superintendent', 'officer-in-charge', 'principal', 'director', 'head of home', and so forth. Not infrequently, domestic work is considered to be a major component of residential work and, in many agencies, ancillary staff will have duties that overlap those of professional workers. For example, in many homes for the elderly and in children's homes, people are employed for combined domestic and treatment functions (e.g. cleaning – 'relief' care workers who substitute for the house mother when she has time off from work).

Professional training for residential work has done little to build public confidence in the enterprise. Nearly all basic professional training courses for residential work have been of one year's duration. With the exception of a few courses established following the publication of the Williams Report, training has been confined virtually to child care where the greatest impact on professional development has been made. The pattern of one year of basic training compares unfavourably to the two years for field social work and three years for teaching and nursing. It appears to bear no relation to either the knowledge or skill requirements of the work. There are, for example, no professional training courses in the United Kingdom that equip a person to implement the concept of 'milieu therapy'. Such training, with its emphasis on the 'daily round and common task' as integral to the total treatment of emotionally damaged children, would elevate the residential worker from his traditional custodial and holding role to that of 'life-space' therapist. Courses started at the Universities of Bristol and Newcastle, in 1960 and 1961 respectively, have done much to promote both the theory and practice of residential child care and to advance the thinking and skills of senior practitioners including those with basic training in other disciplines. However, there are few opportunities of this sort for advanced training in residential work.

Ad Hoc Solutions
Many efforts have been made to recruit adequately trained staff in sufficient numbers for residential work in order to reduce the high turnover of staff, to improve conditions of work and quality of service and to enhance the status of residential workers. Attempted solutions are of three main types. First, there have been many *ad hoc* efforts which often occur in response to critical incidents that generate public disquiet and

official inquiries. The outcomes of official inquiries usually result in renewed efforts of problem-solving that focus on matters like recruitment and training. For example, the establishment of the first training courses in residential child care under statutory auspices followed the recommendations of the Curtis Committee in 1946.[15] Until then, the only training for residential work had been undertaken by voluntary organisations. Another example is the drive to recruit graduates, teachers and others with suitable academic and personal qualifications for housemaster posts in approved school, and the establishment of special training programmes for approved school staff that followed the disturbances at Carlton House Approved School in 1958.

A Separate Profession for Residential Care?
A second kind of effort to upgrade the quality of residential care staff is the work of the Williams Committee[16] which argued that residential care should be developed as a *unified but separate* profession. The Williams Committee, after an exhaustive inquiry into the problems of staffing residential homes, proposed that basic professional training for residential work should be of two years' duration. Its most important recommendation was that training courses should consist of 'a common basis and options to be selected by students in accordance with their special interests and that this shall be the normal method of entry into residential work'.[17] In addition, the Williams Committee recommended the development of one-year courses for mature students who wanted to develop a special career in residential work, and advanced courses for experienced and qualified practitioners.

The Williams Report drew attention to an area of social service that hitherto had been examined only in a piecemeal manner. It also produced some attractive propositions related to the methodology of residential care; in particular it supported the idea that common principles are applicable to residential settings serving a wide range of client groups. However, the recommendations of the Williams Report have never been implemented fully although it did lead to the establishment of full-time training courses for senior staff in homes for the elderly and handicapped.

The failure of the Williams Committee to mobilise resources for the development of a separate residential care profession was partly due to oversimplification of the problematic aspects of the situation. Indeed, the Committee made recommendations for common patterns of training and a separate career structure for residential work in the face of evidence that did not support this policy.[18] Many people believe that, because of the varied objectives sought by residential care institutions and the people who work in them, there could not be as much transferability of knowledge from one setting to another as is envisaged in the

Williams Report. Nevertheless, it is possible that imaginative schemes could be developed to allow students to sample several settings before choosing to work with a client group. This sort of enlarged training experience might result in greater transferability of knowledge and skills from one section of residential work to another. However, this possibility still remains to be explored.

In one respect the philosophy of the Williams Report has been implemented in the development of the Residential Care Association (RCA). The RCA (formerly the Residential Child Care Association) has developed, in large part, as a result of the reorganisation of local authority social service departments which placed different kinds of residential establishments under one administration. The RCA, through its monthly journal, *Residential Social Work*, and an annual review, represents the professional interests of all those engaged in residential work and day-care. This new association is distinct from the British Association of Social Workers (BASW) which in 1974 recognised for the first time a basic qualification in residential work as suitable for membership of BASW.

Residential Work Is a Part of Social Work
The third and most recent type of solution to the problems of developing quality staff for residential care is the recent attempt to integrate residential work into the profession of social work. These important issues are discussed in greater detail in the publications of the Central Council for Education and Training in Social Work (CCETSW) which attempted in 1972 to formulate a policy concerning training for residential work. A working party to expedite this effort was established. The findings of the working party have been published in two stages, in 1973[19] and 1974.[20]

The working party, before it could reach any conclusions about the status of residential work, had to resolve several important issues. One of the first tasks was to identify the range of settings where the social work profession has a major responsibility for the primary care of the residents. This task is difficult because of the diversity of residential practice. The care of even a single client group may be based on the philosophies and treatment methods of different professional disciplines. It is possible to take the view that practice in some settings is a branch of an alternative profession. For example, the residential care of the chronically sick and disabled can be conceptualised as a branch of general nursing practice; the care of former psychiatric patients in rehabilitation hostels and half-way houses as a branch of psychiatric practice; the care of the elderly infirm and the elderly confused as branches of geriatric practice; and so forth.

Any definition of the boundaries of residential social work is probably arbitrary, in part because of the piecemeal development of the services which has resulted in their location in different organisational and administrative systems. The CCETSW working party solved the problem by excluding institutional care that is the direct responsibility of another profession from its remit. However, this solution is, to some extent, unsatisfactory when the problem is studied from another perspective. If the client groups in residential care are examined, we find thousands of children and adults living in psychiatric and mental subnormality hospitals, not because they need medical care and treatment, but because alternative resources are unavailable. However, responsibility for the care of these people, whose needs are primarily personal and social and not medical, lies with staff whose training is in hospital work rather than social work.

Another conceptual problem is raised by the care of children in residential special schools. The daily care of children in these establishments is often the responsibility of teachers and ancillary workers who undertake these aspects of the work as 'extraneous duties'. These staff members do not receive social work training. There are many people who approve of this because they regard the care of the children as an integral part of a total educational process, not as a separate professional undertaking.

A similar difficulty faces the former approved schools, not nearly all of which are administered by local authority social services departments (except in Scotland). These schools have been re-titled 'community homes with educational facilities' in order to emphasise their social and rehabilitative functions, although many of the principals of the schools are not social workers, but professionally qualified teachers. The euphemism 'community homes with educational facilities' clearly illustrates the problem of defining social work boundaries in these types of establishment.

It is by no means a universal assumption that residential work is part of social work at all. Righton states that even in those establishments that specifically provide social services (e.g. children's homes and old persons' homes) as distinct from education and medical services, only recently has the work done by staff been thought of as social work.[21]

Despite these conceptual problems, the CCETSW working party produced convincing arguments for regarding residential work as part of social work. These arguments are summarised as follows: (1) residential work is part of the profession of social work because it holds values, objectives and clients in common with other social work services; (2) its practice requires the same basic knowledge and skill; (3) while some aspects of residential practice may require specialised knowledge and skill, the major differences between residential work and other social work specialisations are technical. Differences between residential care and other types of social work practice are assumed to result from the nature of the professional settings in which residential social workers operate and the modes of interaction that are characteristic of practice in these settings.

These arguments have resulted in the working party's most important recommendation: that there be *a single pattern of training for field and residential social workers*. A majority of the working party recommended that the Certificate of Qualification in Social Work (CQSW) should be the basic qualification for *all* social workers and that there should be, in addition, *two levels of training* with a qualification at each level. Some members opposed the concept of the two-tier training and, in a minority report, proposed that the CQSW should be the only qualification for residential work.[22]

In the Discussion Document,[23] the working party recommended two types of training for residential work: social work training and training in welfare work. The latter training was intended for different categories of assistant staff (e.g. care staff in old people's homes) whose duties are to provide personal care and basic services. Candidates would be awarded a Certificate of Qualification in Welfare Work (CQWW) on completion of training.

The recommendation for a CQWW course was strongly criticised by the social work profession which argued that residential tasks could not be divided into social work and welfare work. Consequently the working party, in the final report, amended the original proposals; but it maintained that training at *different levels of social work* was needed because of the diversity of roles and responsibilities carried by staff in organisations providing residential care. (Readers should note that the CCETSW is not implementing the recommendation made by the working party for two-tier social work training. Instead it is proposing a new form of training, the Certificate in Social Service (CSS), which is intended to meet the training needs of different categories of staff in social service agencies, including some from residential settings.)[24]

RESIDENTIAL WORK *is* SOCIAL WORK

In the final part of our discussion we describe some of the elements of social work practice in residential settings in order to clarify the relationship between residential practice and other social work specialisations. There is great saliency to this issue at the present time, because new training policies for residential work are being implemented during a period when traditional social work practices are also undergoing change. For example, the articulation of a unitary model, which aims to integrate group work and community work with casework, clearly has important implications for residential practice because residential practice is regarded by some to be a separate method.[25] However, readers should note that literature from the USA on social work practice does not refer to residential work as a methodological specialisation.

Objectives
We can state that the goals of residential work are, like any social work activity, to maintain and enhance the personal and social functioning of clients. Thus it is possible to enumerate the objectives of residential work in the short and medium term as follows:

(1) To help clients cope with the painful experience of admission, and of separation from members of family and friends.
(2) To facilitate their adjustment to a new primary living group.
(3) To assist clients in finding solutions to the various life problems that have resulted in their admission.
(4) To enable them to establish contacts with the world 'outside'.
(5) To help them sustain meaningful relationships inside and outside the residential setting.
(6) To prepare clients for 'departure'; whether this means leaving the setting to build a new life in the community, transferring to another residential setting, or, indeed, preparation for death, as in the case of people in terminal care.

Long-term aims are for clients to attain a full and true sense of their own identity and worth, to exercise autonomy and to become fully integrated members of the community, whether or not they continue to live in residential care.

Tasks
'Social work,' states Boehm, 'seeks to enhance the social functioning of individuals, singly and in groups, by activities focused upon their social relationships, which constitute the interaction between man and his environment.'[26] The 'activities' engaged in by residential workers are incorporated in the acts of planning, creating and maintaining an environment for shared daily living. Details of these activities are given by Righton, who states:

'Residential workers provide for residents what the rest of us have to provide for ourselves: food, a bed, a roof, a structure of routines, opportunities for enjoyment of leisure, a framework for feeling secure and exercising freedom of choice; someone to talk to, to test out ideas on, and to try out the limits of behaviour with.'[27]

Thus, in residential work, opportunities for planned intervention are the myriad social situations that constitute everyday living. Much of the worker's day is spent with individuals and groups ('direct' interventions), or in acting on their behalf ('indirect' interventions). Throughout the day he endeavours to balance the needs of individuals with those of the whole group and to balance needs for dependence with strivings for independence. He learns to assess situations accurately and to employ appropriate techniques on the basis of his assessment. He learns when to act promptly, decisively and authoritatively; when to support, sustain and encourage ventilation of feelings; when to provide opportunities for reflection; and when to mediate, negotiate, collaborate, bargain and comfort. And, of equal importance, he learns when *not* to intervene.

The indirect interventions made in residential work are wide ranging. They include: preparations for a single activity on the daily programme; negotiations made on a client's behalf with schools and places of employment; collaboration with field social workers in repairing or maintaining family relationships; bargaining with the administration for resources; and establishing good relationships between the unit and the neighbourhood.

Getting up in the morning is an example of a deceptively simple social situation in which residential staff are involved. For many people in residential situations, young and old, beginning the day is fraught with difficulties. Thus the immediate objective is to help them get a good start to the day. Elderly and disabled people in care often require assistance with the mundane tasks of getting out of bed, going to the toilet, washing and dressing. Their feelings of distress and shame over these disabilities have all to be understood and supported.

For others in residential care, the obstacles are more emotional and social than physical. Whittaker, writing about the residential treatment of emotionally disturbed children, states that the success of an entire day depends on effective management at the beginning. He comments:

'Many of the children we work with in residential settings find morning a difficult task to manage: waking-up, getting out of bed, dressing, getting to breakfast, and getting off to school may be major hurdles for the child to overcome.

'By the time he finally arrives at school he may have been in several fights with peers and a protracted argument with an adult. It is not difficult for us to imagine how the remainder of his day may be hampered by this poor beginning.[28]

It is impossible for us to detail the interventions, 'direct' and 'indirect', that can be made in this situation alone. But, whether it involves people whose fluctuating moods make them depressed, apathetic, withdrawn, fearful and resentful of having to face the day, or whose physical disabilities require them to be dressed and undressed, considerable expertise is required for this apparently simple social operation to be successful.

Every social situation could be examined for its content and dynamics, knowledge and skill requirements. In each situation, the 'instrumental' aspects of the work (i.e. lifting, washing, dressing, recreation) are essentially focal points that enable residents and staff to engage in emotionally significant interactions. To facilitate communication, many modes are used, some verbal, others non-verbal. Different communication patterns have to be understood, interpreted and acted upon by workers. As a result of the transactions in these situations, meaningful relationships that enable residents to work more effectively on their life problems are fostered and cemented.

Routines (of which 'getting up' is but a single example), when skilfully and flexibly managed, are important means of support for residents as they provide reference points around which the fabric of the day is built. The danger in residential care is always that routines are established as ends, instead of means to further ends. Routines and other institutional arrangements provide ready-made defence systems that frequently protect staff from having to grapple with the emotional content of their work. When routines are accredited too much emphasis, the consequences are nearly always dysfunctional. They result in the alienation of residents, who feel their needs are sacrificed to administrative efficiency and expediency.

Any enterprise that aims to meet the total needs of people who are dependent for various reasons, or who require help because of former acts of deviancy, is always vulnerable. The sources of its vulnerability are the intense feelings and excessively inappropriate behaviour patterns that are generated in these settings. To remain in touch with the undercurrents of feeling that pervade the life of a residential unit is extremely difficult. The task requires that workers remain in touch not only with the feelings of group members but with their own as well.

It is regrettable that support and supervision in residential work are neglected subjects. An adequate model of supervision has yet to develop, but the casework model is clearly insufficient to account for the complex variables in the residential situation. Support systems are essential for staff development and as means of obtaining open communication between members of the residential team.[29] Open communication enables staff to appraise their own strengths, weaknesses and coping capacities, and helps them communicate more effectively with clients.

Self-awareness is vital because of the influence of personal feelings and attitudes on professional judgement and decisions in shared 'life-space' situations. The gamut of emotions – feelings of stress, tension, anxiety, love, hate, joy and anger – have to be contained and communicated so that a sharp focus is maintained on the primary task.

The responsibility for ensuring that the unit-as-a-whole is working towards agreed objectives is carried by the head of the establishment and senior staff. The organisational and leadership task includes planning, implementing and co-ordinating individual care and treatment programmes in concert with field social workers and relevant practitioners from other professions. This work involves careful assessment and matching of needs and resources. It requires making effective use of resources available to the unit, inside (i.e. of staff and residents) and outside (i.e. of neighbourhood, educational, and employment systems). In addition, it requires a willingness to innovate and experiment with alternative techniques.

Relationship to Other Social Work Specialisms
In a brief discussion such as this, differences between residential practice and other types of social work practice are easily misrepresented. These differences are largely attributable to varying emphases placed on the activities involved in developing an environment for shared daily living. Readers should not underestimate the special knowledge and skills that are required for residential work, particularly the nurturing skills employed in dealing with the tasks of daily living, and the 'programme' or creativity skills that are required to make full use of opportunities for social education and life-enrichment.

It is also easy to underestimate the special knowledge and skills required for work with different client groups. In child-care practice, primary care is emphasised as the means to assist children's healthy growth and development. Nurturing provision thus provides opportunities for therapeutic intervention with children whose ego development has been incapacitated as a result of earlier emotional deprivation or distorted primary relationships. Special approaches (e.g. in regression) which are not commonly employed in other areas of residential practice are used in this type of work.

Work with school-age children can be contrasted to the work undertaken in 'therapeutic communities' which is based on democratic principles and the sharing of responsibilities. There the nurturing functions of the unit are exercised by the total group of staff and residents. Because there is a different focus in these settings, worker techniques bear more similarities to social group work than to stereotypical residential care.

In the 'therapeutic community' the essential difference between the interventive approach of a residential worker and of a social group worker is his utilisation of the primary processes of daily living as the principal mode of intervention. Social caseworkers, group workers and community workers provide experiences that are additional to, and in association with, clients' ongoing primary life experiences. Their methods have been described as 'associate methods' of helping.[10] The role of the social caseworker and group worker when working with clients in residential settings is similar to their role in other social work contexts. Their efforts supplement and complement the activities of the residential worker operating in the primary sphere.

Effective teamwork is essential for residents to retain and maintain a true sense of identity, and to achieve social integration. Our concept of team includes: professional social work staff working on and through the tasks of daily living; members of related professions involved in the life of the unit, e.g. psychiatrist, psychologist and schoolteacher; administrative, ancillary, and domestic staff; volunteers. All make important contributions to residents' welfare.

Few of the objectives that we have identified for residential work can be reached by residential staff working in isolation. Therefore the team concept must embrace community-based social workers whose collaboration is needed for the attainment of common goals. The conditions for effective teamwork between residential and community-based social workers are discussed by Righton.[31] He states that residential social work is neither so different from other types of social work that there are no overlapping skills, nor so similar that roles are interchangeable. Roles must not only be clearly defined, but understood by all members of the team.

Few dispute that one of the most pressing problems in social work is the quality of relationships between residential workers and their community-based colleagues. Some of the factors affecting the development of a common identity for social workers in these inter-related spheres of practice are discussed by Righton in another of his articles, which is cited above.[32] Ainsworth uses a systems approach to discuss the professional integration of residential work and 'field' social work.[33] Both writers clearly demonstrate the amount of work that remains before a common professional identity can emerge.

We maintain very firmly that residential work requires all the knowledge and skills of social work. Nevertheless we find it difficult to conceptualise residential work as a 'methodological specialisation'. This is in part because of the heterogeneity of residential services. In addition, there is at least one other important reason for considering a 'methods approach' to be a limited perspective. That is, it runs the danger of encapsulating residential work. We would prefer to reject any view that the activities of residential work take place within a closed social system; our view is that residential work is part of an open system which is in continuous exchange with its related environmental systems.

Implications for Training
We believe that an integrated approach will enable professionals to make more effective use of residential settings for the purpose of train-

ing. At present, residential placements are used quite differently in training programmes for field and residential social work. The residential placement in fieldwork training, which is usually no longer than a month, is rarely viewed as an opportunity for skill development. In contrast, training for residential work requires extensive practical experience in a residential situation and the importance of practical experience in other social work settings is sometimes ignored.

It is not always recognised that residential settings provide many opportunities for learning the range of interpersonal skills required for working with individuals and groups. For example, the interventions made by field social workers in crisis situations and the techniques required for coping with angry and violent outbursts from clients can be learnt effectively from practical experience in appropriate 'life-space' settings. In addition, many of the 'specialist' skills required in intermediate treatment are basic skill requirements for residential practitioners.

CONCLUSIONS

In our introduction to this discussion of residential work, we stated that it is impossible to ignore the ambivalence with which our society views residential services. In our discussion we have considered the implications of these attitudes for the development of services, for residential practice and for training. We do not consider the integration of residential practice into the mainstream of social work to be a panacea for the many problems facing residential work. The extent to which the proposed patterns of training increase the proportion of qualified social workers entering residential practice remains to be seen. Many people believe that the majority of residential workers will be forced to take non-CQSW courses because it is not universally accepted that residential work demands the knowledge and skills required for social work. It is also thought that employing authorities will continue to give high priority to recruiting trained fieldworkers and lower priority to having qualified residential staff. It is a paradox that despite the proposals made by the CCETSW for integrated training, those who work in the most intensive of all social work settings are unlikely to receive adequate training for the job. We maintain that *all* residential workers, irrespective of their role in the organisation, require training in social work to equip them for the task. We are thus sympathetic to the minority view expressed in the CCETSW working party report which states that no qualification which is lower than the level of the CQSW should be introduced as a qualification for residential work.[34] However since new training programmes are only just being implemented it will be several years before we actually know the effects of these changes.

Clearly, there is no single solution to the many problems facing those who develop, administer and operate residential services. At the core of the matter is the relatively low value that the community sets upon residential care which determines the functions of, and the resources available for, residential work. As long as resources are unavailable residential centres will continue to emphasise custodial care and protection at the expense of integration and rehabilitation.

In order to emphasise this point, we conclude our discussion with another of Balbernie's observations:

'In a "solid" family the parents become, or can be helped to become, aware of the child's difficulties as an aspect of their difficulties. . . . But in some families, less well grounded, more anxious and uncertain of themselves, more threatened by a deviant child, such insight is often too painful, and such awareness of mutual responsibility not yet possible. The child has then to carry the full projection.'[15]

When a responsible community recognises its own part in the creation of its 'bad objects' and 'sick members', it provides the healing environment and the means for reintegration. In accepting its responsibility society has also to participate in the reintegrative process. Otherwise, like an 'immature family', the 'bad objects' will continue to be pushed 'out there' and to receive the full projection of society's failings. Thus, the concept of integration will remain an illusion.

NOTES AND REFERENCES FOR CHAPTER 12

1 Richard Balbernie, *Residential Work with Children* (Oxford: Pergamon, 1966), p. 3.
2 R. J. Titmuss, *Commitment to Welfare* (London: Allen & Unwin, 1968), ch. 8, 'Community care – fact or fiction?', p. 100.
3 *Tyn-y-Pwll, The House in the Hollow* (Bedford: privately published, 1974).
4 See, for example, H. Polsky, *Cottage Six* (New York: Wiley, 1962).
5 M. Meacher, *Taken for a Ride: Special Residential Homes for Confused Old People, a Study of Separation in Social Policy* (London: Longmans, 1972).
6 P. Righton, *The Continuum of Care: The Link Between Field and Residential Work* (The Barnardo Lecture 1973; Ilford, Essex: Barnado's, 1974).
7 ibid.
8 M. Wolins, 'Group care: friend or foe?', *Social Work* (NASW), vol. XIV, no. 1 (January 1969), pp. 35–53.
9 See, for example, J. Berry, *Daily Experience in Residential Life. A Study of Children and Their Care-Givers* (London: Routledge & Kegan Paul, 1975).
10 M. Oswin, *The Empty Hours* (London: Penguin, 1971).
11 J. Brown and D. Solomon, 'Leisure time interests of children in residential homes', *Residential Social Work*, vol. XIV, no. 8 (August 1974), pp. 246–9.
12 E. J. Miller and G. V. Gwynne, *A Life Apart: A Pilot Study of Residential*

Institutions for the Physically Handicapped and Young Chronically Sick (London: Tavistock, 1972). See also R. D. King, R. D. Raynes and J. Tizard, *Patterns of Residential Care* (London: Routledge & Kegan Paul, 1971).

13 Titmuss, *Commitment to Welfare*, p. 100.

14 CCETSW, Discussion Document: *Training for Residential Work* (Central Council for Education and Training in Social Work, February 1973), ch. 1, p. 3, para. 6.

15 *Report of the Care of Children Committee* (The Curtis Report; London: HMSO, Omd 6922, 1946).

16 *Caring for People: Staffing Residential Homes* (The Williams Report; London: George Allen & Unwin, 1967).

17 ibid., p. 166, para. 23.

18 See for example, ibid., p. 157, paras. 54–6.

19 CCETSW Discussion Document: *Training for Residential Work*.

20 CCETSW, *Social Work: Residential Work Is a Part of Social Work*, Report of the Working Party on Education for Residential Social Work, CCETSW Paper no. 3 (January 1974).

21 P. Righton, 'Two cheers for residential social work', *Southfield Papers*, no. 3 (London: Southfield Trust, 1974), p. 1.

22 *Social Work: Residential Work is a Part of Social Work*, pp. 37–40, paras 230–50.

23 CCETSW, *Training for Residential Work*, p. 26, paras 88–9.

24 CCETSW, *A New Form of Training: The Certificate in Social Service*, CCETSW Paper no. 9:1 (1975).

25 The CCETSW working party defined residential work as: 'a method of social work in which a team of social workers operates together with a group of residents to create a living environment designed to enhance the functioning of individual residents in the context of their total environment'. CCETSW, *Training for Residential Work*, p. 15, para. 50.

26 Werner W. Boehm, *Objectives of the Social Work Curriculum of the Future* (New York: Council on Social Work Education, 1959), p. 54.

27 Righton, 'Two cheers for residential social work', p. 1.

28 J. K. Whittaker, 'Managing wake-up behaviour', in A. F. Trieschmann, J. K. Whittaker and L. K. Brendtro, *The Other 23 Hours* (Chicago: Aldine, 1969), ch. 4, p. 120.

29 See J. Berry, *Daily Experience in Residential Life*.

30 H. W. Maier, *Child Care as a Method of Social Work* (New York: Child Welfare League of America, 1963), pp. 62–81.

31 P. Righton, 'Cooperation between community-based social workers and residential staff', in *Residential Care and Treatment* (Advisory Council on Child-Care, Keele University Conference Report, July 1970), pp. 25–39.

32 P. Righton, *The Continuum of Care: the Link Between Field and Residential Work*.

33 F. Ainsworth, 'The uneasy integration', *Residential Social Work*, vol. XIV, no. 3 (February 1974), pp. 66–9.

34 CCETSW, *Social Work: Residential Work Is Part of Social Work*, p. 40, para. 249.

35 Balbernie, *Residential Work with Children*, p. 2.

PART III

ISSUES AND PROBLEMS IN EDUCATION
AND PRACTICE

In this last part we attempt to describe some of the major issues that will be encountered in efforts to integrate social work methods. In Chapter 13, 'The incomplete profession' by Neil Gilbert and Harry Specht, a distinction is drawn between *direct practice* (or social work), which is concerned with providing services to individuals, families and groups, and *indirect practice* (or social administration or social welfare), which is concerned with the management, maintenance and change of the institution of social welfare. Gilbert and Specht take the position that the profession will be 'incomplete' so long as educational institutions and the organised profession do not recognise this distinction and alter patterns of professional training to take account of it.

In Chapter 14 we deal with some educational issues. We start with the assumption that choices in education for social work cannot be made without taking account of society's needs for social work manpower. Models of social work education must be selected, at least in part, on the basis of these needs. Education that relies upon a too highly integrated model of practice, we argue, may *not*, at this time, be the model of choice for training most social workers in the United Kingdom.

In the final chapter of the book we summarise the major issues and problems that have been discussed throughout the text. These are problems of communication and choice.

Chapter 13

THE INCOMPLETE PROFESSION *

Neil Gilbert and Harry Specht

The profession of social work is incomplete: it has developed a commitment to services but has failed to develop a commitment to welfare.
This incompleteness is one reason for its difficulty in responding effectively to demands placed on it by a society in transition and upheaval.

This diagnosis of the state of the profession is not original. It follows
a recurrent theme on the duality of social work practice, played under
different titles throughout the profession's history. In 1905 Richmond
wrote of the 'wholesale' and 'retail' methods of social reform: in 1929
probably the best known and most enduring variation was composed by
Lee under the title of 'cause' and 'function'; in 1958 Burns spoke of the
distinction between 'social work' and 'social welfare'; in 1963 Schwartz
discussed the 'service' and the 'movement'; and in 1972 Richan identified different underlying language systems in social work.[1] And this is
only a partial list.[2]

While duality still exists, in recent years its nature has changed substantially. The balance has shifted from services to welfare, and the
consequences are now filtering into the field with results disappointing
for the profession's commitment to both welfare and services. The purpose of this article is, first, to examine this shift and the adjustments that
have been made and, second, to propose a course of action designed to
fulfil a substantive commitment to welfare while maintaining the integrity of social work's commitment to services – not to mitigate but to
invigorate the duality inherent in social work practice.

In this discussion the authors refer to *services* as the specific and concrete activities that professionals engage in to assist those in need. They
include all direct-service activities such as therapy, counselling, education, advocacy, information gathering and referral. Such activities are
the major concerns of casework, group work and those aspects of community organisation in which direct services are provided to community
groups and organisations.[3] These activities will be discussed collectively

* Reprinted from *Social Work* (NY), vol. XIX, no. 6 (November 1974) with
permission of the authors and the National Association of Social Workers.

as social work services and direct services and the professionals engaged in them will be referred to as social work specialists and direct-service workers.

Welfare, in the framework of this chapter, deals with the professional activities that focus on both change in and maintenance of the institution of social welfare. *Institution* in this instance refers to the system of programmes conducted by public and private agencies that have the express purpose of providing mutual support for individuals, families and groups.[4] Professional activities involved in social welfare include indirect services such as planning, policy analysis, programme development, administration and programme evaluation. The social welfare specialist does not deal directly with those in need, but rather focuses on the institutional structure through which those in need are served. These activities will be referred to as indirect services and social welfare, and the professionals engaged in them will be referred to as indirect service workers and social welfare specialists.

SERVICES AND WELFARE

Sixteen years ago, in 'Social welfare is our commitment', the keynote address to the National Conference on Social Welfare, Burns described the difference between the two commitments and provided the framework for developing the profession's other side. Burns indicated that the conference had changed its name from 'social work' to 'social welfare' because social work had come to signify only 'certain categories of people who are involved in our social service', those with 'a specific series of skilled services'.[5] She stated that there was nothing undesirable about the professionalisation of certain types of social welfare activities, but that the term 'social work' focused too narrowly on professional functions. 'Social welfare', on the other hand, 'seemed most comprehensively to embrace the entire field of social welfare and the concerns of all those who were interested in it regardless of their functions, professional orientation, skills, and affiliations'.[6] Ironically, the table of contents of the conference proceedings listed Burns's address as 'Social work is our commitment'. The profession of social work appears to have little understood and been little affected by her lucid and instructive charge.

This result was not entirely unforeseen; Burns identified three obstacles to the fulfilment of social work's commitment to welfare. First, the technical skills and knowledge required to affect the structure of welfare services were in short supply in social work. Second, social workers perceived themselves as lacking the influence and political power needed to affect public policy decisions. Third, the profession had no commitment to a cause.[7]

A significant proportion of social workers today have a surfeit of commitment to causes and no longer suffer from a lack of belief in their political acumen. In contrast, there has been little development of the knowledge, skill and technical expertise that Burns thought necessary for fulfilling a commitment to welfare. But in the process of change, the commitment to services has been drastically diluted, if not completely erased, as resources, practice skills and knowledge designed for the service enterprise were stretched and twisted in efforts to accommodate new departures. Rein's observation in 1970 is much to the point.

'Individual social workers may, of course, function as reformers in the areas of employment, income distribution, and political power – but these activities are marginal to their professional tasks. In this sense they are professionals who are radical rather than members of a radical profession.'[8]

How did all this come about?

IMPULSE FOR CHANGE

Social work's commitment to services was made at the beginning of this century. At that time, as Austin points out, strategies for societal change were rejected in favour of a concentration on services:

'Particularly significant in the conflict between these two approaches was the decision made in 1910 by the board of directors of the New York School of Philanthropy to concentrate on the training of caseworkers for direct service positions in charity agencies. In doing so they explicitly rejected the recommendation . . . that social workers should concern themselves with the issues of public policy rather than with the provision of financial assistance on a case-by-case basis. . . . The practitioner-oriented curriculum which the New York School adopted, built around the personnel needs of locally based individual and neighbourhood centered programs, was to become the model for all schools of social work until the 1960s.'[9]

In the early 1960s, along with the general national impulse for social justice, social work was gripped by an impulse to make social welfare an instrument to deal with societal inequities. Social workers' belief systems and orientations were profoundly affected by three developments: (1) the civil rights movement, which was part of and probably the cause of a general revolution in human relations, (2) the evolution of national programmes such as the War on Poverty and Model Cities, which were directed at producing large-scale social change, and (3) the growing concern at the start of the 1970s with questions of institutional inequality.[10]

The social work profession, as Austin notes, became the whipping boy for the advocates of institutional change because social casework failed to develop effective means for dealing with poverty:

'The high point of the assault was the speech by Sargent Shriver . . . in 1964 announcing that there was no place for casework in the war-on-poverty programs. . . . The attack on casework and the organized social work profession continued throughout the [War on Poverty] together with strong support for the principle of using nonprofessionals and generalists rather than social work specialists as staff in community action programs. This attack which was also supported by many professional social workers was so successful that the membership of the professional association voted in 1969 to overturn the principle established . . . in the 1920s that social work was a distinctive profession based exclusively on a systematic program of professional education at the graduate level.'[11]

With individual services suffering a crisis of confidence, how did the profession express the impulse for social justice? One might say that it attempted to deal rather with injustice, but in poor form. The National Association of Social Workers, the Council on Social Work Education and schools of social work and social welfare were not prepared with a substantive, distinctive means by which social work could address problems of poverty, discrimination and inequality. An impulse is not a commitment but only a feeling pushed on by energy without any direction. Demonstration, disruption, confrontation – the tactics of Saul Alinsky based on the idea that 'power is all' and the tactics of the civil rights movement – were adopted by many social workers as behaviours of choice for committed professionals.

Caught short, social workers used the only means available to the profession at the time for responding to demands for change – its services.[12] Many concluded that casework was not effective for any purpose, and those who provided services to clients in need began to address themselves politically to social problems. Custodial care, institutionalisation, supportive services and clinical intervention were to become almost anathema in the social services – all seen as variations of 'blaming the victim'. Attention and resources were devoted to protest activities, street people, social action and manifestations of social ferment like drug abuse, sexual liberation and new forms of communication. Many practitioners attached themselves to causes that were written in the day's headlines and that changed almost as frequently.

The authors attended a recent meeting of social workers, called to discuss with the school's faculty what professionals in the field believed the school should teach. As the list of problems having priority grew longer and wider in range, one professional who works with the state senate inquired, 'Is there any problem that you think you cannot deal with?' He then said he finds it difficult to convince the senate – a legislative body reasonably sensitive to the concerns of social welfare – that social workers can do *anything* well. Apparently this sentiment is not peculiar to the California state legislature. The Family Service Association of America issued the following statement:

'It will be impossible for graduates to be prepared for [direct-service-giving] positions if the school has set an educational goal for them that is too general and has encouraged them to place no value on working with the individual predicaments and life problems of people. . . . Many students do not achieve in graduate schools of social work a fundamental grasp of [the competence needed for case-work practice]. They do not develop a commitment to, or even an awareness of, the need for working with and for individuals and families. They do not emerge with an adequate theoretical base for practice in usable form.'[13]

The social work profession responded inadequately to the impulse for change because the training, skill and knowledge required for a sustained and meaningful commitment to welfare were lacking. Social workers enthusiastically rushed to engage themselves in one new programmatic arrangement after another with little to show for the effort either in social change or increased knowledge and competence. All the heat did not forge a commitment to welfare, but rather served to consume the substance on which the commitment to services is based.

SEARCH FOR UNITY

Many factors internal and external to the profession influenced its response to the social forces at play since the 1960s. One internal factor of central concern to social work educators was that the profession's perennial search for unity hampered change and the development of a commitment to welfare.

Many have long considered that the duality of social work practice is a source of strain within the profession. Proposals for mitigating this strain generally have been couched in terms of unity, which would seem desirable. Indeed, unity is an objective hard to resist in almost any context (man with man, man with nature, nation with nation, husband with wife). The problem is not the objective, but the means proposed to achieve it in social work.

Achieving unity has been equated with mixing the educational elements required to produce the direct-service practitioner and the social welfare specialist. For instance, there are proposals to create the generic social worker by fusing service and welfare commitments into a single function, such as the mediating one described by Schwartz.[14] Levin proposes 'a social policy base for unifying the component sequences of the curriculum and for shaping their content'.[15] And Richan suggests that the unifying elements may be found in developing a common professional language.[16]

The common thrust of most of these proposals is towards achieving unity by creating a core curriculum in which direct-service practitioners and welfare specialists mingle in the same core courses. The degree to which the identities, skills, knowledge and practice orientations of the two groups are fused depends on the extent of the core curriculum.

These proposals tend to ignore or at least do not directly address another meaning of unity that has to do with the distinction between mixing and linking. *Mixing* implies creating a new whole by fusing separate identities of constituent elements. *Linking* implies creating a new whole by connecting separate identities of constituent elements.

A UNIFIED SINGLE FUNCTION

In response to proposals that there should be separate systems of social work education for direct-service practitioners and social welfare specialists, Schwartz states the argument for a unified single function – the unity-through-mixing orientation – as follows:

'To create a "department" for each would in fact *institutionalize* the very evils they mean to solve. The "clinicians" would be shielded from any further pressures to bring weight of the experiences with people in trouble to bear on the formation of public policy; and the "social planners" would be set free from the realities of practice and left alone to fashion their expertise not from the struggles and sufferings of people but from their own clever and speculating minds. . . . The planner who has not practised will be as shallow in his policy-making as the practitioner who has not made his impact on policy will be in his work with people.

'Thus the question for the profession is whether it now gives itself over to the polarization of the individual and the social, building it into its very structure, or tries to see more deeply into the connections between the two so that it may create a single vision of the professional function.' [italics added][17]

Schwartz raises an important issue. Is it possible to prepare professionals who can carry a commitment to welfare without first becoming skilled direct-service practitioners? Can they plan for, administer and evaluate services if they have not been directly engaged in providing them? One way to put this issue to rest is to point out that much significant work on social welfare policy, programme, administration and research and evaluation is by non-social workers or those with little direct-practice experience. Among these, to mention a few, are Eveline Burns, Frances Piven, Nathan Glazer, Daniel Moynihan, Edwin Witte, Arthur Altmeyer, Herman Somers, Mollie Orshansky, Wilbur Cohen, Sar Levitan, Gilbert Steiner and Robert Lampman – all welfare experts known for work they have done skilfully, with compassion and commitment. No one knows or cares whether they have mastered the 'conscious use of self' that is legitimately expected of the direct-service worker.

DUALITY OF THE PROFESSION

Another approach to this issue recognises that the profession of social work is, in reality, divided into two branches. In actual day-to-day practice, professionals are clearly engaged in either direct or indirect services, carrying out a commitment to services or a commitment to welfare. If social workers ignore this reality, they are merely leaving it to others to fulfil their commitments. As long as the profession does not fulfil its commitment to welfare it will not have a serious handle on its own future. If social workers are to deal with social welfare, then educators and social planners had better begin to build the programmes and the professional support system that will encourage them to do so.

The call to arms should not be so thunderous as to drown out the practical wisdom of those who caution against polarisation of the profession. When Schwartz stated that 'the question for the profession is whether it now gives itself over to the polarization of the individual and the social', this implied division and disaffection between competing elements in the profession. But another outcome might be possible: separate functional identities that are complementary and mutually supporting might be developed. However, the duality in the profession has manifested itself more in division and disaffection than in complementarity and mutual support.

The rejection of Schwartz's proposition that the planner or welfare specialist who has not practised will be 'as shallow in his policy-making as the practitioner who has not made his impact on policy will be in his work with people' does not mean that the authors favour the complete separation of the welfare specialist and the social work practitioner nor that they condone either one's ignorance of the other's line of practice. On the contrary, to the extent that each knows and understands the other's practice, his own grasp of the profession is enhanced and the profession benefits from the support each provides the other. The question is one of substance and degree. The goal is the development of separate functional identities within the framework of a unified profession.

IMPLICATIONS FOR EDUCATION

The search for unity may be summarised in terms of the following four broad models of social work education: the generic model, integrated core model, linkage model and independent model. (See Figure 3.)

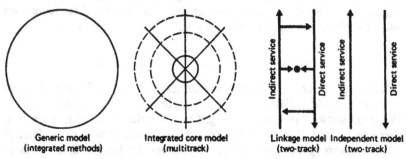

Figure 3 Educational Models for Integrating Social Services and Social Welfare

Generic Model

Essentially, this model – which represents the extreme of unification through mixing – prepares professionals for direct service to individual clients, families or groups. In some instances students will have courses in community organisation and social planning. This type of programme produces professionals whose major commitment is to service and who have a good deal of information about organisations, planning and welfare systems. Frequently professionals so trained know a little bit about a lot of things but are not well enough versed in the practice requirements or any specific area to offer a substantial contribution to either service or welfare.

Clearly, a commitment to services is important and worthy of professional development. But it is not the same as a commitment to welfare, nor should it be. Those who want to provide direct services to people, whether through therapy, counselling, advocacy or leisure-time activities, are obligated to master relevant knowledge and skill about inter- and intrapersonal interventions, group dynamics, social and individual pathology and professional behaviour in working with clients, agencies and other professionals. Attempting to expand their functions to include all types of social intervention and social change efforts can only have deleterious results. Their professional equipment is likely to be a thin patchwork quilt. Training for a commitment to services should aim to produce professionals who are as highly skilled as possible at what they do.

Two-Track Independent Model
At the other extreme, the two-track independent model calls for a clear separation in developing professional practitioners for welfare and service functions. One track trains for clinical practice (direct services); the other trains for social planning, research and administration (indirect services).[18] The distinctive feature of this model is that training for one functional track is so independent of training for the other that an entire school of social work may specialise in either area. There is no reason why both tracks must be located in one school and, if they are, there is no curriculum requirement that forces students and faculty of the two tracks to intermingle.

As the authors see it, neither the generic nor the two-track independent model seems likely to train satisfactorily both types of workers within the framework of a unified profession. The generic model attempts to provide a framework for unity by mixing practice functions so thoroughly that, in the process, service and welfare commitments are diluted. The two-track independent model attempts to produce substantial commitments to service and welfare, but in so doing introduces sharp separations and divisions that increase the likelihood of polarisation.

Multi-Track Integrated Core Model
In this model the various tracks may be found under the traditional labels of casework, group work and community organisation; micro-system, mezzo-system and macro-system; or direct and indirect services. Or they may focus on problem areas such as community mental health, ageing and child welfare. The integrated core of these educational programmes may vary in size from a few courses to a substantial part of the curriculum (at which point this model takes on aspects of the generic one). Usually the integrated core includes, at a minimum, courses in human growth and development, research and social policy, in which students from all tracks mix. These core courses are designed, first, to provide students with a body of knowledge relevant to the pursuit of their various lines of practice and, second, to provide the academic binding for unification within the school and profession. Thus they offer a substantive answer to the question: what is it that unites these various specialists in one profession?

Compared to the curriculum for training direct-service practitioners, the programmes for indirect services are relatively new to schools of social work and generally not as well formulated. This is not to suggest that all is well with the direct-service training or that the area does not need new curriculum developments, experimentation and change.[19] However, the focus of this discussion is on curriculum requirements for indirect services. The following four major areas in which the social welfare specialist must have expertise suggest the depth and complexity of the knowledge base for the curriculum of the multi-track model:

(1) Problem analysis. This includes skills in research, data collection and interpretation of findings to reveal linkages between causes and problems; and assessment of needs and resources.

(2) Programme design. This includes skills in organisational analysis and understanding of alternatives in the construction of service delivery systems; skills in budgeting, cost-benefit analysis, and other forms of systems analysis such as the planning-programming-budgeting system (PPBS); and planning for co-ordination and resource acquisition.

(3) Development of and work with decision-making systems. This includes political organisation and processes; uses of priority-setting schemes, organisational operations and knowledge and skill in the structuring of planning and administrative agencies; and the acquisition and promotion of needed technical support (e.g. for economic development, therapeutic programmes or manpower training).

(4) Evaluation. Like the first area, this includes skills in research and data collection but also calls for political and organisational skills. The function of evaluation differs from problem analysis in terms of its objective, which is to enable the community to determine the extent to which social service programmes meet their goals.[20]

The authors see a crucial distinction between the essence or core of the welfare specialist's practice orientation and that of the direct-service practitioner. With the understanding that any effort to extract the essence of phenomena as complex as the skill and knowledge base of social work practice must in some measure simplify reality, the differences may be stated as follows:

* The core practice orientation of the direct-service worker deals with individual and group problem-solving methods, drawing upon social-psychological interpretation and relating mainly to personal and interactional variables.

* The core practice orientation of the indirect-service worker deals with the methods of applied social research, drawing upon empirical interpretation and relating mainly to structural and organisational variables.

By requiring students in both the direct- and indirect-service tracks to take the same set of courses, the integrated core model tends to emphasise the objective of professional unity at the cost of functional relevance.

Two-Track Linkage Model

What and how much knowledge should be shared by direct- and indirect-service workers? The main distinction between the integrated core model and the two-track linkage model is the manner in which this issue is addressed in the curriculum. Both models might include, for example, research, policy analysis and human growth and development courses for the direct and indirect services. In the integrated core model the substance of these courses would be the same for the direct and indirect services. These and perhaps other courses are, in effect, what form the integrated core. In the two-track linkage model the substance of these courses would be different.

Although it is not the authors' intent to design a curriculum, they will attempt to convey a sense of how this model might be put into operation. Consider, for instance, the research requirement. In the indirect-service track, planning and evaluation of social welfare programmes are among the skills that must be mastered. Students in this track would take research courses designed to maximise these objectives; students in the direct services, in which the knowledge of applied research methods is less central to practice, would take a substantially different type of research course, designed mainly to produce intelligent consumers or users.

The responsibility for creating the linkage, for teaching direct-service practitioners something about the practice of the indirect services and how they might collaborate with social welfare specialists, falls to the indirect-service instructors. Similarly, it would be the responsibility of instructors in the direct-service track to develop, for example, special courses designed to give social welfare specialists an understanding of the nature and requirements of practice in the direct services. Precisely what courses would fall in each track and the most appropriate points for creating linkages are matters open to detailed analysis and experimentation.

There is another type of course in which students from both tracks might intermingle. This would be a course dealing with the history of the profession and its role in developing the institution of social welfare. Such a course would highlight what it is that unites these two types of specialists in one profession – their common interests in the problems, issues, clients and programmes of social welfare and the complementary skills they bring to bear on them.

Finally, there is the question of the kinds and degrees of specialisation that an MSW programme designed according to the two-track linkage model might have. There can be a wide variety of arrangements for specialisation within each of the two major tracks.

CONCLUSION

Recently, a number of schools of social work have developed programmes for training professionals for social welfare, which suggests that
the field may be attempting to fulfil its dual commitment.[21] But the
appearance of these programmes causes a high degree of uneasiness in
the profession, and opposition may be expected from a number of
sources. What seem to be some of the bases for opposition to a commitment to welfare?

A commitment to welfare entails an abstract, reflective and long-range
outlook. As Burns notes, such a commitment is 'a state of mind which
conceives of one's own job as part of a wider whole and where attention is focused always on the wider objective'.[22] This approach is at
variance with that of the political activists, who are more inclined toward immediate action and engagement in the current struggle rather
than toward the deliberate study and systematic evaluation that mark a
commitment to welfare.

The current ideological demands of minority faculty, students and
practitioners for curriculum emphasis on the Third-World perspective
of racial minorities involve a narrower and more particularistic outlook
than that required for the training of welfare specialists. This struggle
between the universal and the particular is an important one in the
profession. It is related to the problem of finding the proper balance
between our commitments to services and welfare only because it has
emerged out of the same historical currents. However, it is a different
and, as Hughes notes, perennial problem:

'This strain . . . is found in some degree in all professions. . . . The
professional may learn some things that are universal in the physical,
biological or social world. But around this core of universal knowledge there is likely to be a large body of practical knowledge which
relates only to his own culture. . . . While professions are, in some
of their respects, universal, in others they are closely ethnocentric. In
fact, inside most professions there develops a tacit division of labor
between the more theoretical and the more practical; once in a while
conflict breaks out over issues related to it. The professional schools
may be accused of being too "academic"; the academics accuse other
practitioners of failure to be sufficiently intellectual.'[23]

The debate over the appropriate balance between general knowledge
and group-specific knowledge in which the social work profession is
now engaged will no doubt continue, along with the search for unity
between direct and indirect services. However, the latter search deals
with a different dimension of professional development which constitutes

a strain in all professions, as Hughes also notes: 'Every profession considers itself the proper body to set the terms in which some aspect of society, life or nature is to be thought of, and to define the general lines, or even the details of public policy concerning it.'[24] That is, every profession must come to grips with the problems created by its duality of commitments.

A third and potentially the strongest source of opposition is from the direct services. Direct-service practitioners have taken quite a battering. Seemingly endless studies demonstrating the ineffectiveness of casework – coupled with a decade-long assault on services by the social action–community organisation–social planning–social policy analysis axis – have devastated them.[25] Coming after the collapse of the 'grand illusion' of casework's bright future contained in the service amendments to the Social Security Act in the 1960s, it is no wonder that in the 1970s direct-service practitioners are anxious about their place in the field. From their viewpoint, welfare specialists are 'the enemy'. The notion of complementary and mutually supporting functions may be unpersuasive in light of these experiences. On the contrary, there is deep-seated concern in the profession that the development or our commitment to welfare will require giving up our commitment to services.

Given these various strains, is it possible for social work to develop the capacity to fulfil a commitment to services and a commitment to welfare to become a complete profession? Perhaps, but such developments await the best efforts that social work professionals have to give. Social workers might begin by ceasing the useless and debilitating attacks on one another, reaffirming the profession's commitment to offering services of high quality, and seeking ways to foster the development of the profession's other side. A reassessment of educational models for the purpose of enhancing the functional integrity of services and welfare within a unified professional framework may be a useful first step in this direction.

NOTES AND REFERENCES FOR CHAPTER 13

1 See Mary Richmond, *The Long View* (New York: Russell Sage Foundation, 1930), pp. 214–21; Porter Lee, *Social Work as Cause and Function and Other Papers* (New York: Columbia University Press, 1937), pp. 3–24; Eveline Burns, 'Social welfare is our commitment', *The Social Welfare Forum, 1958* (New York: Columbia University Press, 1958); William Schwartz, 'Small group science and group work practice', *Social Work*, no. 8 (October 1963), pp. 39–46; Willard C. Richan, 'A common language for social work', *Social Work*, no. 17 (November 1972), pp. 14–22.

2 For a concise review of the variations on this theme, see William Schwartz, 'Private troubles and public issues: one job or two?', *The Social Welfare Forum, 1969* (New York: Columbia University Press, 1969), pp. 22–43.

3 Community organisation (CO) does not fit neatly into the distinction between service and welfare activities. CO practice, as Rothman points out, may be categorised under locality development, social planning and social action. Locality development is mainly concerned with service activities, and social planning with welfare activities, but the social action model seems to contain the potential for both types. See Jack Rothman, 'Three models of community organization practice', *Social Work Practice, 1968* (New York: Columbia University Press, 1968), pp. 16–47.

4 For a more detailed explanation see Neil Gilbert and Harry Specht, *Dimensions of Social Welfare Policy* (Englewood Cliffs, NJ: Prentice-Hall, 1974).

5 Burns, 'Social welfare is our commitment', p. 4.

6 ibid., p. 3.

7 ibid., pp. 15–19.

8 Martin Rein, *Social Policy* (New York: Random House, 1970), p. 297.

9 David M. Austin, 'The anti-poverty wars of the 20th century', unpublished paper (Waltham, Mass.: Florence Heller School for Advanced Studies in Social Welfare, Brandeis University, 1972), p. 10.

10 For a thoughtful analysis of the impact of these changes in one city, see Alfred Kahn, 'Do social services have a future in New York?', *City Almanac*, no. 5 (February 1971).

11 Austin, 'The anti-poverty wars of the 20th century', p. 33.

12 See Harry Specht, 'The deprofessionalization of social work', *Social Work*, no. 17 (March 1972); Don C. Marler, 'The nonprofessionalization of the war on mental illness', *Mental Hygiene*, no. 55 (July 1971); James D. Orten, 'Political action: ends or means?', *Social Work*, no. 17 (November 1972).

13 Family Service Association of America, 'Position statement of family service agencies regarding graduate schools of social work' (New York, 1972; mimeographed).

14 Schwartz, 'Private troubles and public issues', pp. 36–43.

15 Herman Levin, 'Social welfare policy: base for the curriculum', *Social Work Education Reporter*, no. 17 (September 1969), p. 40.

16 Richan, 'A common language for social work'.

17 Schwartz, 'Private troubles and public issues', pp. 35–6.

18 For descriptions of this kind of practice, see Bartlett, *The Common Base of Social Work Practice*; Goldstein, *Social Work Practice*; Pincus and Minahan, *Social Work Practice*.

19 For an example of what some of these changes might look like, see Rein, *Social Policy*.

20 For additional discussion, see Burns, 'Social welfare is our commitment', pp. 9–12; and Gilbert and Specht, *Dimensions of Social Welfare Policy*, pp. 9–12.

21 For example, see programme statements of School of Social Work, University of Washington; School of Applied Social Sciences, Case Western Reserve University; School of Social Work and Community Planning, University of Maryland; School of Social Work, University of Minnesota.

22 Burns, 'Social welfare is our commitment', p. 21.

23 Everett C. Hughes, 'Professions', *Journal of the American Academy of Arts and Sciences*, no. 92 (Fall 1963), pp. 661–8.

24 ibid., p. 657.

25 For example, see *Social Service Review* (entire issue), no. 46 (September 1972); Fischer, 'Is casework effective?', *Social Work*, no. 18 (January 1973), pp. 5–20.

Chapter 14

USE OF UNITARY MODELS IN EDUCATION FOR SOCIAL WORK

Anne Vickery

Our brief account in Chapter 3 of the Pincus/Minahan and Goldstein unitary models shows that they do not attempt to integrate all of the knowledge required for casework, group work and community work into one mode of practice. Their purpose is to conceptualise the generic knowledge and skills that all social workers should have. Broadly speaking they provide, first, a structural view of all the social phenomena with which social work is concerned, which includes the social worker and the change system and an account of the dynamic inter-relationships between parts of the whole structure. Second, they provide an account of the process of planned change and the problem-solving or learning process that is fundamental to all social work practice. Third, they provide an account of the social work skills that are held in common by all social workers. The question for us is, how useful is it for the training of social workers?

It may be helpful to delineate two distinct uses of the unitary model:

(1) *As a perspective on social work practice as a whole*: Teaching might concentrate on the most prominent feature of the model which is its structural view of all the social phenomena with which social work is engaged including individuals, families, groups, organisations and communities. In addition, there may be teaching about general processes of planned change and problem solving, and identification of the skills that are common to all social workers. This use of the model might be considered an essential beginning of training for all kinds of workers. Although much more detailed additional knowledge would be required for the worker to practise effectively in his chosen area of specialisation, the unitary model would, nevertheless, provide him with a clear understanding of how that specialisation related to the entire field and how he himself should relate to the whole.

(2) *As a vehicle for training workers to practise more than one method*:

additionally, teachers might use the model to integrate methods that might otherwise be taught separately. In the United States there are an increasing number of schools of social work at which integrated methods courses are taught. Typically, they combine casework, family therapy and group work. Sometimes they include aspects of community work such as work with community groups. In comparison with the use of the model as a perspective, these courses have to devote far more detailed attention to teaching processes of planned change and problem solving, and more time is devoted to development of the skills required to practise with a range of methods. With regard to the structural aspects of the model, students have to acquire precise knowledge of a range of social systems; minimally, this requires knowledge about individuals, families and groups; optimally, it includes knowledge about organisations and communities as well.

THE UNITARY APPROACH AND THE METHODS SPECIALIST

Before discussing these two uses of the unitary model, it will be useful to compare the kind of practitioner that the unitary model is intended to produce with the kind of specialised methods practitioners that other models are intended to produce. Following this, we can deal with the question of what kind of practitioner is needed both now and in the future.

The unitary model emphasises the need for a practitioner who is able to assess problem situations on a broad canvas, to detect the need for intervention outside the client-system, to be a more active 'go-between' in mediation between client groups and social institutions. This does not mean that the individual practitioner must be competent to intervene in all of the social systems concerned in a particular problem situation. But it does require the ability to judge what kind of expertise is needed, who should be involved, and the capacity to work in collaboration with variously oriented practitioners, consultants, administrators and paraprofessionals.[1]

To compare this kind of practitioner with the specialised methods practitioner is to risk making inaccurate generalisations. Nevertheless, we think that the content of training influences the way in which the student develops, and that a too-exclusive emphasis on specific areas of knowledge is bound to create a narrow perspective. The arguments in favour of a unitary model often give a vivid picture of the kind of specialised 'methods' practitioner that the model is not intended to produce. Generally, the type of worker that is eschewed is the traditional caseworker, family therapist and group worker rather than the community worker. The 'undesirable' professional is perceived to be highly skilled in face-to-face encounters with the kind of client with whom he has been trained to deal, and as one who places great emphasis on the efficacy of these encounters to bring about a desired change in the client system. This emphasis is thought to diminish interest in environmental problems because it frequently obscures the need for intervention in systems other than the client and does not encourage the practitioner to consider whether the problem might be better dealt with by a method other than the one in which he is specialised.

Many specialised methods workers would, rightly, reject this description of their work, for in reality their practice demonstrates the breadth described in the previous section.

Nevertheless, some practitioners have attributes associated with the more traditional specialised methods worker. We have mentioned that, with the development of knowledge and skill in casework, there was a degree of distortion in social work practice because some areas of skill were developed at the expense of others and some aspects of practice were devalued. The same imbalances may occur in regard to the newly developing practice of community work. That is, emphasis may shift to the environment with a consequent neglect of the individual. When these kinds of imbalances occur, social problems tend to be defined in ways that suggest that the kind of intervention in which the worker is especially skilled is in fact the most appropriate form of intervention for that particular problem. The caseworker will define problems as residing in the individual; the community worker will perceive that problems are caused by societal institutions.

WHAT KIND OF PRACTITIONER IS NEEDED?

The drive to train practitioners who can assess problems broadly and can intervene flexibly is, in part, a reaction to this last state of affairs. But this trend toward generalism brings with it the danger of encouraging the training of a professional who 'knows a little about a lot of things'.[2] In other words, it supports the idea of a professional who lacks the skills of the specialised methods worker and who is therefore incapable of being effective in situations in which those skills are needed, such as in situations in which family treatment or group work might be the method of choice, or long-term casework with a severely disturbed person. But to be aware of this danger is not to argue against broader frames of reference for basic professional training.

Rather, it forces us to turn to the question of the manpower needs of the field and the likely effects that various forms of training will have on these needs. Ideally we should try to have the best of both alternatives. That is, the professional should have special knowledge and skills available to help in situations where they are required along with a capability, however specialised, to assess problems differentially and to promote intervention in and among a wide variety of systems. However, there is a difference between the kind of practice for which most students are currently being prepared and the kind of practice they will, ideally, need to undertake in the future.

There is always a tension between the view that training should support the current methodological practices of agencies and the view that training should be a powerful force for improving agency practice. This tension has been especially acute in recent years because of the expectation that training should equip most students to work with the whole range of local authority clientele. This expectation clearly influences the curriculum and guides the skill development of students in fieldwork placements.

Currently the majority of social work students will, in fact, be employed by local authority social services and social work departments. Here, they deal in the main with individual clients and families. They will be responsible for delivering concrete statutory services and initially will have little time and freedom to be methodologically innovative. Despite the current growth of interest in group work, family therapy and community work, the methods that are still most used in local authorities are provision of information, advice giving and casework with a strong emphasis on material provision and/or social control. Although the newly qualified worker's knowledge about practice with different kinds of client problems will be variable, he will know enough about the legislative framework of his service and the resources of his agency and community to bring the client and available resources (including his own skill) into some kind of creative relationship.

However, the general development of thinking in relation to practice is moving away from the idea of the professionally trained worker being prepared only for this individual kind of work with clients. This movement has several different aspects. Here, we want to discuss the increasing use of para-professionals, the greater emphasis in social work on environmental intervention, the need for special knowledge and skills and changes in the way social workers are deployed.

THE PARA-PROFESSIONALS

The increasing use of social work assistants, case aides and volunteers has had several effects on the professional worker's role. Naturally, much depends on the type of work performed by the para-professional but, generally speaking, any or all of the following effects may occur. First the professional may be freed from work that does not require professional training. Second, some tasks may be better done by the para-professional (e.g. befriending the isolated elderly, discharged prisoners and grossly deprived families); the professional may have to accommodate to being less skilled than the para-professional in performing some tasks. Third, para-professionals usually need some kind of supervision, preparation, consultation and support that should be provided by professionals. Tasks have to be allocated to workers trained at different levels with an understanding of the respective roles of each in relation to clients.

INCREASED EMPHASIS ON ENVIRONMENTAL INTERVENTION

As we have already noted, most social workers have always been sensitive to the importance of clients' material needs and community resources. Nevertheless, intervention in the environment and the role of the social worker as advocate, mediator and broker has been given more attention in recent years. Unfortunately a worker's desire to influence a client's environment often outstrips his capacity. The theoretical side of these aspects of practice is less well developed than aspects of practice designed to help clients improve their coping capacities. Moreover, the aims of environmental intervention have recently become more ambitious. It is not always easy to acquire resources to which clients are legally entitled. But currently it is suggested that workers should be active in policy change and development of new resources. This is usually beyond the scope of the majority of posts that newly qualified workers occupy.

The limits of this scope are clearly evident in Goldberg's study of social work with the aged in a London borough welfare department. At the fieldworker's level of operation certain features distinguished the work of trained workers from that of untrained workers. Perhaps the most important was that the trained worked more closely with medical agencies, statutory departments, voluntary agencies and volunteers. Because of this they succeeded in bringing more items of practical and medical help to their clients. At this level the study shows that failure to obtain certain items of practical help was often due to slowness of administrative procedures and to deficiencies in the services both within and outside the welfare department.[3] However, it was beyond the scope of the social workers to do more than report and record these deficiencies. For some items, part of the remedy lay with managerial staff and part with the local authority committee members. An example of one deficiency was lack of transport for the elderly to get to clubs and day centres in which the borough had invested considerable resources.

Goldberg writes: 'It seems important to bear in mind the interrelationships of the various parts of the welfare services. A great expansion of one part – additional social workers or clubs – may be less beneficial in the long run than a more modest but balanced, expansion of all interrelated parts of a service which would put its resources to optimal use.'[4] This is precisely the view of social services that a systems approach encourages. But the good sense of Goldberg's observation is misleading if it conveys to the reader the belief that the remedy is easily obtained. Accounts of service developments usually show the need for the developers to understand, consult with, and reconcile the aspirations of, a wide range of interested parties holding diverse and conflicting views.[5] The social worker dealing with lack of transport has a responsibility to mediate for change within his own agency. But in a large and complex department, having made the case for change, the social worker with individuals and families must probably leave it to others to influence the resource providers. Cheetham and Hill discuss how local authority community workers can influence change:

> 'The effective influence of community workers in local authorities will depend very much on how far the structure and organization of large departments follows an "organic" model which expects professionals at all levels in the hierarchy to contribute to decision-making and policy formulation. This is one of the most critical problems facing Social Service Departments with implications for all social workers, not only community workers.'[6]

Additionally, the ability of social workers to influence change will depend on their knowledge of *how* to intervene in their own organisation and *how* to influence other organisations. An integrated methods course would, theoretically, teach the knowledge and skill required for intervention in 'change-agent systems' and 'target systems outside the client system and action system' as well as in 'client systems'.[7]

THE NEED FOR SPECIALISED KNOWLEDGE AND SKILL

The emphasis of the unitary approach on assessing problems on a very broad canvas should not obscure the need for adequate knowledge in specific fields. A recent study of the problems of the relatives of people with schizophrenia shows the failure of some social workers to understand the problems with which they were dealing.[8] Similar failures are reported in work with relatives of handicapped children and adults.[9]

Gaps in knowledge and expertise can be discovered in other fields of practice such as welfare rights, delinquency, marital work, child abuse and sexual deviance. If basic professional training were to maintain a generalist approach in relation to fields of practice then specialist knowledge would need to be developed post-professionally. Also, if skill development in methods can be taken only a short way in basic training, then there is a need for some workers to specialise later in methods that require considerable supervised experience such as marital and family therapy, behaviour modification, certain forms of group work such as with disturbed adolescents and deviants, and work with community groups.

Another dimension of specialised practice relates to the work of para-professionals, who are likely to be more specialised in terms of the kinds of clients with whom they work and to have more circumscribed tasks than the professional social worker.[10]

IMPLICATIONS FOR THE ORGANISATION OF FIELDWORKERS

Although at present the majority of basic grade professional workers are doing a large part of the direct work with individuals and families, it is certain that with current developments in the field their role in future social services will be different. The generalist professional is more likely to have a mixture of roles such as enabler and co-ordinator of teams of para-professionals; the collaborator in, and sometimes the co-ordinator of, multi-disciplinary teams; the mediator between client groups and service organisations; and the resource developer. He will need to be skilled in assessing problems of a general nature and in planning interventions. The specialist professional is likely to be some of all these things, but compared with the generalist worker he is likely to do more face-to-face work with client groups who have special difficulties and who require specially skilled forms of intervention; this worker will also offer more consultation to other workers on special aspects of practice. How can all of these roles, knowledge and skills be brought together so as to ensure that client needs are properly met?

Several writers recently have discussed the differential use of staff. Many point up the need for teams of workers who combine a mixture of knowledge, skills, interests and personalities. The teams need to be small enough to inter-relate in some depth and large enough to provide a mixture of abilities needed by the consumer population.[11] How teams should be organised to employ their para-professional or assistant workers is still an open question. Organising principles include allocation of responsibility by task, by types of 'cases' and by episodes of service.[12] All of the principles require that the professional worker be a good diagnostician as well as a planner and co-ordinator of interventions.

It is important to note that in many of the published case studies illustrating and analysing multi-methods and unitary approaches, the workers are apparently free to focus their attention and energy on one specific unit or problem such as on the inhabitants of one tenement building or the population of one prison; or in a wider geographical area on a particular kind of clientele such as young people or psychiatric after-care patients.[13] Two conditions appear to be crucial to any degree of success. One is that the workers have adequate knowledge of all the social systems that impinge on the clientele; the other is that the workers are able to organise themselves for particular purposes into cohesive teams and to carry flexible roles.

KNOWLEDGE OF THE SOCIAL ENVIRONMENT

Regarding adequate knowledge, there is clearly a limit to how much one worker can know. Knowledge of all the relevant social systems needs to be much more specific and locally based than the kind of general knowledge that workers would normally have about organisations such as schools, hospitals, tenants' associations and social security offices. It must be as detailed and personal as the knowledge a caseworker has about a particular family. This kind of knowledge is only acquired by regular contact with, and study of, the social systems and the people concerned. Therefore, in any geographical area, some division of labour needs to be worked out in relation to building up that knowledge. Methods for storing and making it available to workers have to be established.

This is probably the task of the workers with more managerial responsibility. The more comprehensive the service of the agency, the more difficult the task is likely to be. No matter what people's over-riding difficulty, they are all exposed to a wide variety of social systems, any of which might be a target for intervention. Nevertheless certain key social systems tend to cluster round certain problem areas so that the wider the range of problems with which the agency deals, the larger the number of systems involved. The generalist workers may have to relate in rapid succession to a community home, a school and a youth club about a child; then to a psychiatric hospital, a day centre and a voluntary organisation about an adult schizophrenic, and so on. This worker needs access to information acquired by quite prolonged contact with these agencies. This is easily achieved by a worker covering a very small geographical area,[14] but impossible for a worker covering a larger one. The information has to be built up by a number of workers and made available to him within his agency or his network of working relationships.

The more specialised the service, the less difficult the problem of adequate local knowledge is likely to be. Examples of the kind of teamwork we are discussing seem to derive mostly from agencies and services with a particular focus such as family service agencies, and psychiatric and geriatric services. But in addition to knowledge of formal organisations, it is important to have equally good knowledge of informal local networks and community groups.

WORKING RELATIONSHIPS

With regard to the second crucial condition (the need for cohesive work groups and flexible working relationships), the degree to which different workers can collaborate is dependent on several factors: freedom from tasks that are outside the concern of the team; security and ability to share with colleagues; a high degree of agreement on values, goals and strategies; and a high degree of understanding of each worker's responsibilities and abilities. The physical presence of workers with different methods specialisations in one agency does not, by itself, ensure integrated approaches. Even the development of integrated working relationships between social caseworkers and social group workers in a small agency requires considerable effort.[15] Additional difficulties arise in interprofessional relationships. Only day-to-day collaboration under skilled direction is likely to resolve misunderstandings over the respective functions, knowledge, expertise and roles of different workers.[16] Thus the integration of interventions requires not only the desire for unitary work, but time, resources and discretionary freedom are equally important.[17]

INTEGRATED APPROACHES AND ISSUES IN TRAINING

We have attempted to give a brief account of the kinds of practice in which professionals may be engaged in the future. To summarise, they will require skills to do the following: to assess problems and plan interventions at a generalist level; to co-ordinate the efforts of a variety of workers including para-professionals; to judge when and how to use specialist workers; to intervene within their own organisations and in other organisations; to organise the collection and dissemination of adequate information for effective practice; to collaborate with a wide range of people, including professionals who are not social workers; and to contribute effectively to policy formulation. We now have to consider how the unitary model can aid in the preparation of this kind of generalist.

In the United Kingdom, discussion of the educational objectives of social work training is confused by uncertainty about the boundaries of social work practice.[18] Referring to our previous discussion of direct and indirect services and to Gilbert and Specht's article, 'The incomplete profession', an examination of most basic courses would indicate that they prepare practitioners only for direct services. Academic preparation for work in the indirect services such as the acquisition, management and planning of resources, and policy formulation and research has been associated traditionally with the discipline of social administration. However, many professional social workers do in fact move by way of promotion into managerial posts that involve the planning and creation of new resources, inter-organisational work, and the influencing of policy. Currently there is no insistence on special training for these jobs. But given the increasing complexity and size of the personal social services, it is clear that the profession has to concern itself with preparation for this kind of work.

The unitary model of social work practice implies the integration of direct and indirect professional functions. The reasons why such an all-embracing objective of basic professional training is neither helpful nor feasible are already clearly delineated by Gilbert and Specht. Nevertheless, it is important to avoid making too rigid a dividing line between the direct-service and indirect-service practitioner. In what we have said about practice in a direct-service agency, we clearly envisage social workers being in the 'middle range' of practice, playing strong mediating and advocacy roles in relation to indirect-service practitioners;[19] and we also envisage the inclusion of 'grass roots' community work within the methods used by direct-service practitioners.

If professional social workers are to acquire the qualities we have outlined they will need in their basic training some preparation for use of intervention methods with a variety of resource systems such as their own agency, other agencies, informal community groups and neighbourhoods. However, it may not be possible for a worker to become a truly competent methods generalist through basic professional training alone. Goldstein argues that the competent generalist is a 'specialist' in the sense of needing a training that makes high intellectual and academic demands.[20] Courses in this country must be adaptive to the intellectual needs of social work students who have varied educational backgrounds. It would be unwise to generalise in detail on how unitary models should be used. Already, many courses are teaching a unitary approach, and it remains to be seen which kinds of student can benefit from greater or lesser degrees of exposure to it.[21]

In principle, we would argue that in basic training unitary models should be used to provide the unitary perspective of the generalist practitioner, and to encourage skill development in as wide a variety of modalities as may be practised with beginning competence. But, like Goldstein, we believe the course must offer opportunities for specialisation in terms of problem area. He writes:

'I do not think, at this point in time, a total generalist programme is possible or feasible. . . . An educational programme may have a generalist orientation insofar as it attempts to educate students to the generic knowledge and an organic conception of social problems that undergirds all of practice. But, at some point, it should offer the opportunity for the kinds of learning that will yield the knowledge and skills that are required to prepare these students for the effective execution of their own capabilities.[22]

THE UNITARY PERSPECTIVE IN ASSESSING AND PLANNING INTERVENTIONS

In the United Kingdom many basic professional courses attempt to extend methods teaching beyond casework by having separate sequences in the other methods. This does not have the same effect as an integrated methods sequence in which students are taught to assess human situations by using varied frames of reference. For example, class discussion of a case of an unsupported mother living in a slum and who is suspected of child neglect is likely to be different in an integrated methods sequence than in a more traditional casework or group work course. Students with a theoretical background in social systems will deal with concepts of mother–child relationships, maternal deprivation, stigma, poverty and squalor, kinship and community relations, and service systems. It might be argued that such a wide-ranging discussion is not useful because it will not help the student decide what is to be done. However, more narrowly focused case discussions that centre, for example, on family dynamics or the psychopathology of an individual attract the same kind of criticism. By contrast, when more wide-ranging considerations are brought to bear, it is easier to identify something in the configuration of social systems that *can* be changed, thereby having some effect on the problem, however modest. Experienced students typically identify a large number of things needing attention at different systemic levels. This opens up the possibility of discussing what needs to be done and what can be done, and the extent to which the skills required for forming relationships and implementing interventions at one systemic level can be transferred to another level.

This use of the unitary model is designed to develop the student's analytic cognitive skills in assessing complex problems and outlining plans for intervention. It does not assume that the students should personally implement the plans, but rather that the student is preparing to contribute to the work of a team such as we have already described. This use of the model, as a perspective in problem assessment, seems to be an essential ingredient in the core training of all professionals, no matter what field of practice they are preparing for and what methods they will be using initially. Even minimal exposure to the unitary perspective is likely to enhance a student's motivation to develop skill in collaborating with other workers.

INTEGRATED SOCIAL WORK METHODS

Apart from the use of the model as a perspective, we want to comment on its use in teaching a course that trains a worker to practise a variety of methods. Here the identification of common skill areas becomes crucial. These areas can be expressed in a variety of ways. One rationale for training workers in both casework and group work is that there are really only two modalities for the worker's interactional skills. He relates either to an individual such as a troubled parent, a magistrate, a housing manager and a committee chairman; or he relates to groups such as a group of troubled parents, colleagues, a family group, a community group, a committee. However, this is not to suggest that if the student is taught social casework and social group work he will be capable of implementing a unitary approach and intervening in the wide range of target systems that a unitary model encompasses. It is important to distinguish knowledge and skills needed by a worker who can offer clients alternative service modalities, and the knowledge and skills needed to intervene in systems other than the client system. It is not only the size of the client system that demands a particular set of skills, it is also the purpose of the worker's interaction in target systems of all kinds. Here the expression of various skill areas in terms of roles becomes helpful. While relating directly to clients and action systems, workers may be in roles such as enabler, teacher or therapist. While relating to other target systems, workers may be more often in roles such as broker, mediator, advocate or adversary. These last have very different implications from the first for worker activity, and require a different knowledge base.

One of the many problems that social work teachers must resolve is how great a variety of practice modalities and social work roles the integrated models can usefully teach. American social work teachers have been experimenting with integrated methods courses for several years, and continue to do so.[23] As we noted earlier, they tend to be confined to the methods of the direct-service worker, and that may or may not include work with community groups. It is difficult to avoid being seduced by arguments that favour a continuing expansion of the student's horizons. In the United States, Briar has described how, as new problems emerge in society, and as social work takes on new tasks, more and more new subjects are added to the generic curriculum. None of them replaces the old subjects or makes them redundant.[24] In Britain we have certainly experienced and still are experiencing the same pressures.

If the standard response to these pressures is to add new content to the curriculum then there is an increased possibility that the student will not learn any one area of practice really well. Knowledge-in-depth is likely to be developed only in the distant future of the student's career when, it is hoped, he will develop expertise through practice. But he may not. Unless the student knows what it means to have studied a subject in depth and acquired some mastery of it, he does not appreciate what he has yet to learn. Briar believes that the inevitable consequence of a too inclusive curriculum would be:

'. . . that our graduates would learn less and less about more and more and we would generate generic dilettantes who can dabble superficially in everything and work deeply and expertly in nothing; over the long run, perhaps the highest price we would pay for this state of affairs is lack of respect for specialised expertise that will accompany the feeling that one has been trained to do anything and everything. However, without a respect for expertise we shall surely behave foolishly. While expertise does not guarantee wisdom, ignorance does insure folly. . . .'[25]

CONCLUSION

In discussing the use of unitary models in training, we have drawn two broad distinctions (i.e. use of unitary methodology as a perspective and metaphor, or its actual use in practice). But in effect we are talking about a continuum between a partial use and a more complete use. To suggest that basic professional training should aim at only a partial use is not to diminish the importance of unitary models. On the contrary, we think they reflect changes in social work education that are responses to changes in the field and in the way social work ought to be practised. The models challenge social work educators to be specific about the kind of practitioner they aim to train and to find an optimal use for a unitary approach.

NOTES AND REFERENCES FOR CHAPTER 14

1 In discussing practitioners we are including practitioners in residential settings as well as those in field settings. In his chapter on residential social work Chris Payne takes the view that it is not a separate method. It should be noted that there is a similarity in the position, functions and abilities of the professional social worker in a residential setting and the kind of professional social worker that we conceive of for a field setting. He works in a team of variously oriented and specialised workers. He has a supervisory responsibility for some. He must be versatile in using a variety of methods. He has to work with and manage relationships in a wide variety of social systems that are external to his setting and that include his local community. We would maintain that a student in a generic course who opts to specialise in residential work is not opting to become a methods specialist but, rather, facing head-on all the problems of a generalist methods worker. At the same time, inherent

in his setting, is a requirement to be expert in the special problems of its particular population, be it children, the elderly or handicapped adults.

2 Gilbert and Specht, *The Incomplete Profession.*
3 Goldberg, *et al.*, *Helping the Aged*, p. 116.
4 ibid., pp. 194–5.
5 See, for example, D. V. Donnison, V. Chapman *et al.*, *Social Policy and Administration* (London: Allen & Unwin, 1965), ch. 8.
6 Juliet Cheetham and Michael J. Hill, 'Community work. Social realities and ethical dilemmas', *British Journal of Social Work*, vol. III, no. 3 (Autumn 1973), p. 345.
7 Pincus and Minahan, *Social Work Practice*, ch. 3.
8 Clare Creer, 'Living with schizophrenia', *Social Work Today*, vol. VI, no. 1 (3 April 1975).
9 Michael Bayley, *Mental Handicap and Community Care* (London: Routledge & Kegan Paul, 1973); CCETSW, *Social Work: People with Handicaps Need Better Trained Social Workers*, CCETSW Paper no. 5 (1974).
10 CCETSW, *A New Form of Training; The Certificate in Social Service.*
11 Robert M. Rice, 'Organizing to innovate in social work', *Social Casework* (January 1973).
12 Donald Brieland, Thomas Briggs and Paul Leuenberger, *The Team Model of Social Work Practice*, Manpower Monograph No. 5, Syracuse University School of Social Work (1973); Carol Meyer, 'Approaches to the differential use of staff', *Social Work Practice: A Response to the Urban Crisis* (New York: The Free Press, 1970), ch. 7; Edward E. Schwartz and William C. Sample, *The Midway Office* (New York: National Association of Social Workers, 1972).
13 See, for example: Purcell and Specht, 'The House on Sixth Street'; Elliot Studt, 'Social Work Theory & Implications for the Practice of Methods', *Social Work Education Reporter* (June 1968); Spergel, 'A multi-dimensional model for social work practice'; T. Fisher, N. Nackman and A. Vyas, 'Aftercare services in a family agency', *Social Casework* (March 1973), pp. 131–41.
14 David Thomas and Henry Shaftoe, 'The patch system: does casework need a neighbourhood orientation?', *Social Work Today*, vol. V, no. 16, pp. 483–6.
15 Lorna Walker, 'Bradford FSU Mothers' Group; group work with the inarticulate', *FSU Paper No. 1*, pp. 22 and 24.
16 Matilda Goldberg and June Neill, *Social Work in General Practice* (London: Allen & Unwin, 1973), pp. 32–5.
17 For a discussion of the working of a multi-method agency, see Michael Laxton, 'Some aspects of developing a multi-method agency', in *Time to Consider* (London: FSU Bedford Square Press, 1975), ch. 1.
18 CCETSW, *Social Work: Setting the Course for Social Work Education, 1971–73*, CCETSW Report No. 1 (1973), p. 20.
19 Hartman, 'The generic stance and the family agency'.
20 Howard Goldstein, 'A unitary approach—implications for education and practice' in F. Ainsworth and J. Hunter (eds), *A Unitary Approach to Social Work Practice*, Conference Report (Dundee: School of Social Administration, University of Dundee, 1975), pp. 33–45.
21 For an account of the conceptual base of one such course, see Jim Jones, *Giving Shape to Social Work* (Association of Teachers in Social Work Education, 1975).
22 Howard Goldstein, 'A unitary approach—implications for education and practice', p. 37.
23 See, for example: Charles Garvin and Paul Glasser, 'The bases of social treatment', *Social Work Practice, 1970*, National Conference on Social Wel-

fare (New York: Columbia University Press, 1970); Whittaker, *Social Treatment*; Kay Dea (ed.), *New Ways of Teaching Social Work Practice* (New York: CSWE, 1972; contains separate papers by Catherine Papell, Lola Selby and Jack Stumpf).

24 Scott Briar, 'Flexibility and specialisation in social work education', *Social Work Education Reporter*, vol. XVI, no. 4 (December 1968), pp. 45-6, 62-3.
25 ibid.

Chapter 15

ISSUES AND PROBLEMS IN UTILISING
A UNITARY METHOD

Harry Specht

In the previous chapters we have devoted a good deal of space to describing various approaches to the development of a unitary method of social work practice. If any reader started out with the impression that it was a relatively simple matter, he is probably convinced by our discussion of historical trends, uses of theory, the types of content to be integrated and educational issues that we do not perceive this to be a simple matter. But we remind readers that it was our intention to expose them to a variety of ideas, some of them contradictory, and to make these complex matters appear as complex as they are. Having done that, we must now address *the* essential question which has probably been nagging the thoughtful reader since he picked up this volume: will a unitary method of social work practice result in a more effective kind of social work?

Alas, in answering this question we shall have to fulfil our earlier promise to equivocate. On the one hand, it should be apparent that a unitary social work method will increase the worker's cognisance of the choices available to him and that it will facilitate communication among professionals who are carrying out a wide variety of functions in many different settings. As we stated earlier, these are two of the criteria by which to judge the utility of theory for practice. On the other hand, however, the final test of the utility of theory can only be made in practice by determining whether clients are better served and whether services are able to achieve their objectives more readily by use of one theory as compared with another. By these criteria it would have to be recognised that the results on unitary method are not yet in nor likely to be available for quite a while. Over the next few years we can expect that educators will attempt to teach and practitioners will attempt to implement a unitary form of social work practice. Preliminary efforts in the local authority social services departments indicate that there are many problems that will be encountered in doing this.[1] In this concluding section we should like to describe the kinds of issues that will be encountered as social workers attempt to resolve these problems.

A generation ago, C. Wright Mills savagely attacked social systems theory for many reasons, one of which was that it is so 'grand' as to be obscure and irrelevant: 'The grand theorist in fact sets forth a realm of concepts from which are excluded many structural features of human society, features long and accurately recognised as fundamental to its understanding.'[2]

From the point of view of social workers the concern about social systems theory is that we may not see the trees for the forest; that it is so high a level of generalisation as to put practitioners out of touch with the phenomena with which they deal – phenomena they might better understand by use of more middle-range theory.

We shall attempt to illustrate some of the benefits and hazards of utilising a higher level of theoretical generalisation with some examples. The following is an excerpt from Pincus and Minahan's discussion of the tasks and strategies of the worker in problem assessment:

> 'Social workers engage in various *activities* in carrying out the *functions* of the profession. . . . Activities and *tasks* to suit the needs of the specific situation being dealt with must be chosen to facilitate these functions. . . . Social workers' activities can be characterized under one of three *approaches* to *intervention* . . . called *education, facilitation,* and *advocacy.* . . .
>
> 'The education approach covers a *cluster of roles* such as those of the *teacher, expert* and *consultant.* . . . This role cluster operates within the *general stance* of *collaborative relationships.*'[3]

We have italicised a large number of the terms in this short passage to draw the reader's attention to the wide range of concepts that Pincus and Minahan use in their description of a unitary method. This particular passage, we believe, is a good example of language that describes common elements in social work practice. Certainly, it would be difficult to identify the language with any one particular methodological or functional specialisation. This common language, we think, is a distinct improvement for social work.

However, problems occur when we leave the level of generalisation at which Pincus and Minahan are working in the above passage and attempt to move to a level of thought that is closer to actual practice. For example, Pincus and Minahan define the concept of 'relationship' as 'an affective bond between the worker and other systems operating within a major posture or atmosphere of collaboration, bargaining, or conflict'.[4] Thereafter in their book they discuss the various practice aspects of relationship in terms of 'collaboration', 'bargaining' or 'conflict'. Now, this kind of reductionism is not any great favour to the practitioner, despite the fact that its concreteness and specificity is attractive. To discuss relationship in these terms is to use a middle-range political science theory that is helpful in understanding only a limited range of phenomena. It is most powerful in analysis of organisational and community behaviour, of less use in understanding small groups, and of little use in dealing with inter- and intrapersonal behaviour. This sort of misuse of middle-range, more specific theory illustrates one of the problems that will be encountered with great frequency as practitioners attempt to operate with a unitary model of social work practice.

Compare Pincus and Minahan's discussion of this concept with the following brief excerpt from Howard Goldstein:

> ' "Relationship" is a somewhat amorphous concept which eludes definition in that it refers to a human phenomenon marked by affective and attitudinal characteristics. We may categorize the relationship by such labels as "good", "dependent", or "intense", but these do not capture its experiential meaning. Its pivotal significance is in its potentiality for providing a climate for change, growth, and confirmation. Perhaps a major measure of the depth and meaning of any relationship is the extent to which it authenticates those who are part of it.'[5]

With that as an introduction he goes on to provide the reader with a rich understanding of the empirical knowledge available about the concept of relationship as well as an appreciation of the mysteries of, and the gaps in, understanding of the concept. Goldstein begins with *general* systems theory and does not rush too quickly to specifics. However, Goldstein's rigour is not without its costs. The latter part of his book is devoted to an explication of a model of practice that is developed deductively from his theoretical framework. However, it proves to be a difficult task to move to a lower level of theory (i.e. to discuss the *specifics* of practice) in a limited space and therefore his description of a unitary model of practice is abbreviated, underdeveloped, and difficult to follow. In this case, the details might better have been left for another book. Thus, although Goldstein's model is theoretically consistent, it is, of necessity, compressed and attenuated.

Pincus and Minahan are much freer and more eclectic in their use of theory. At the conclusion of their chapter in this volume (Chapter 5) they describe their quite flexible approach:

'The model is not based on any one substantive theoretical orientation, such as learning theory, ego psychology, communication theory or conflict resolution, but allows for the selective incorporation of such theoretical orientations in working with specific situations. The social work model for practice is clearly differentiated from any substantive theoretical orientations being utilised. In many practice models the two become so intertwined that the theoretical orientation appears to dictate the purpose of the social worker's practice.'

Thus, the rigorous use of theory, as exemplified by Goldstein, requires a high degree of systematic control and attention to detailing theoretical propositions and empirical verification. More flexible and eclectic use of theory, as exemplified by Pincus/Minahan, may lead to reductionism and oversimplification.

To summarise: we think that a unitary method will enhance the ability of social workers to communicate with one another and with others about their work *at a high level of generalisation*. However, it is extremely important that social workers do not assume that because they have a language that allows them to discuss *some* aspects of practice in common terms, that all conceptual differences among practice specialisations are no longer of use. To the contrary, in the early stages of development, a common language will offer only a small vocabulary and we must not too quickly discard our 'native tongues' which may be richer and more evocative in expressing the ideas and meanings that generated them. 'Transference', 'cohesion', 'resistance', 'authority', 'anxiety', 'catharsis'; these are very rich concepts. If we use them with discrimination, only where they have 'fit', they will continue to enrich our conceptualisation of practice long after a unitary approach is established.

CHOICE: A REVISIT TO THE HOUSE ON SIXTH STREET

A unitary approach to social work practice broadens the perspectives of the professional and vastly increases the number of choices he has. When one deals with a social problem with this perspective there are many possible client systems, many possible action systems and many possible modes of intervention. 'The House on Sixth Street' illustrates this.[6] Although one individual mother comes to the agency for help, the workers find that among the possible client systems are the mother, all of the families in the tenement, other groups living in tenements suffering from the same problems, the landlords, and so forth. Throughout the experience the action system consists, at different times, of the caseworkers who were originally involved, community organisers, lawyers, the tenants and others. In the course of working with the problem the workers use casework, group work, community organisation and several other kinds of interventive techniques. The case history that is told here is very stirring, even exhilarating.

However, one of the reasons why the story is exhilarating is that there seem to be no bounds to what the change agent system (Mobilisation for Youth) was prepared to do to deal with this particular problem. Purcell and Specht note that this particular situation did not require them to be concerned about 'a correct definition of interacting social systems or of the social worker's choice of methods and points of intervention'. Being an experimental and well-funded agency with a very broad brief, they were able to bring enormous resources to bear. Even so, at the end of the paper, the question of choice is framed but not resolved; the authors write that 'The problems that remain far outweigh the accomplishments'. Thus, even this agency's apparently limitless resources were not so limitless as to achieve a satisfying solution to the problem. The breathtaking scope of the action seems to stop us from asking pertinent questions such as: would it have been better to concentrate all of these resources on one aspect of the problem rather than try to deal with them all? were some of the interventions contradictory and did they, therefore, cancel one another out? was this the wisest way for the change agent system to use its resources from the point of view of the agency's long-range goals? who made the choices in the situation, the clients, the workers or the agency? and, was the responsibility for making choices appropriately distributed?

Of course, these questions about choice will arise in regard to efforts to deal with any social problem. They are likely to be much more acute when resources for action are not as abundant as they were in the House on Sixth Street situation. Using a unitary perspective, the worker will be confronted by a panorama of choices for clients, action systems, modes of intervention and change agent systems. He must decide what to do about this panorama of possibilities and at the same time take account of his own limited resources and responsibilities as well as the agency's limited resources and responsibilities. A unitary approach, therefore, does not make the question of choice a simpler one for the worker. Rather, it makes it more difficult. We said in an earlier section that a unitary approach will expand the worker's perception of the kinds of choices available to him. However, the unitary approach to practice enhances the worker's ability to assess problems on a broad canvas far more than it enlarges his capacity to prescribe a course of treatment; while it enlarges the possibilities vastly, *it does not tell the worker what to do*, and for that reason it makes his life more complicated than it is when he uses a more circumscribed and limited methodological approach.

The enlarged perspectives provided by the models described by Bartlett, Pincus/Minahan and Goldstein create problems of choice that extend beyond the problems of selecting theory and knowledge for practice. That is, they confront the practitioner with many possible causes of problems and innumerable possibilities for intervention. How are the choices for action to be made and who makes them? Both Goldstein and Pincus/Minahan deal inadequately with this question. Social choice (i.e. of intervention methods, of programmes, of benefits and of means for financing and delivering them) is a matter in which professional social work interveners play only a small part. These kinds of choices are made via the political, social and market processes that operate in the larger society. These processes are the subject matter of the related content area of social welfare policy which has never enjoyed a very central place in the social work curriculum, nor captured the interests of most social workers. However, the work of Goldstein and Pincus/Minahan is bound to make the study of social welfare policy more germane and alive to the social work practitioner. Without a grounding in social policy concepts and processes, unitary practice will be even more hopelessly adrift than current practice is.

Certainly, social workers must be wary of the fact that a unitary approach confronts the practitioner with so many complicated decisions that the client may easily be pushed out of the choice-making process. This is well illustrated in the Pincus/Minahan text where, on page 241, after lengthy discussion of processes and methods, the authors suggest that 'It *may help* the action system if members are involved in a diagnosis of the system's problems of functioning.' (Italics added.)

The client's primacy in the decision-making process – an important feature of classical social casework – is bound to be undermined by a more complex and technical methodological approach. In utilising any one of the social work methods of old (e.g. casework, group work), the client was dealing with narrower, more circumscribed and more easily understood practices. With a unitary method, the client 'buys' a service that is far more difficult for him to understand; the management of the process is, therefore, more likely to be taken out of his hands. The dangers of undermining the value of self-determination are great; professional social workers will find it difficult to keep in sight the value-based principle that method is to be selected on the basis of what the client wants as well as what the worker's goals are.

A related problematic feature of systems theory is that while it provides social workers with an orientation that is much broader than presently used middle-range theories (e.g. 'role theory', psychoanalytic theory), it is generally more mechanistic than the psychologically based theories. It is better suited to analysis of organisational and institutional behaviour than of individual behaviour. While, at the moment, this may be a useful corrective to a social work practice that has been too much focused on people's inner lives, in the long view it may encourage practice that is insufficiently sensitive to individual needs and problems. It does sound more *avant garde* and progressive to use theory that constrains us to take account of the environment and to understand how institutions impinge on individuals and affect their behaviour. But it may also cause practitioners to neglect the uniqueness and individuality of people in need. People are not 'systems' in the same way that organisations and institutions are. They have inner lives, hopes, dreams and a past. They are much more difficult to understand than organisations which are only symbols and concepts. Thus, systems theory may provide an appropriate framework for the intellectual task of selecting theory and knowledge for practice but it by no means makes practice simpler or easier.

With all its limitations, it is important to bear in mind the great contribution that social casework has made as a means of dealing with social problems. To wit: social casework conceives of a person as being a *unique* and *whole* being in interaction with his environment. A social systems approach can be very useful in providing a framework by which to organise knowledge to understand the *person* in the *situation*, the whole being in interaction with his environment. However, if the effect of systems theory is to focus all attention on the situation, on the external, on the environment, then social work will be in a new kind of imbalance. Social work must relate its efforts at environmental planning, organising, administering, and social action to its unique concern for helping *persons* to effect healthy and constructive social relationships. A too-generalised approach to social change will put social workers into wasteful competition with other change agents like city planners, politicians and trade union organisers.

SPECIALISTS OR GENERALISTS?

Does a unitary approach require that every social worker undertake a systems analysis of each of the problems he encounters in his work? Does the worker have to take account of the 'total' system each time he tries to help a client? Obviously not. Systems theory does not require that we assume that we know nothing about human behaviour and that each experience must begin afresh with a complete analysis of all of the systems and sub-systems that bear upon a problem. Similarly, a bio-social approach to human problems does not require that every proposition in the theory be applied to the case. As we noted earlier, theory is a guide to practice and only useful to the extent that it helps the practitioner to organise his thoughts and help him to keep track of knowledge. In the artful practice of social work, the professional develops skill at being able to sort out problems quickly, at knowing which ones require less or more attention than others, and which ones he has dealt with many times before and which ones are unusual. Therefore, although social systems theory encompasses a wider range of social phenomena than others, with experience and skill practitioners will come to use it as a guide to practice.

However, other models of practice such as casework and group work are more focused on the behaviour of an individual practitioner than is the case with a unitary model of practice: that is, even though the descriptions of unitary practice à la Pincus/Minahan and Goldstein seem to talk about *the* practitioner, they are nonetheless describing 'change agent system' rather than a specific practitioner. The composition of this system is, of course, variable, depending upon the situation. It might consist of an individual, a team, different workers acting in serial fashion or a collection of specialists. Specialisms might be based on different kinds of in-depth expertise and/or different degrees of the same expertise. Vickery deals with some of these questions elsewhere,[7] and we have outlined some of the characteristics of an agency offering unitary approaches (Chapter 14).

These are questions that will be answered only as efforts go forward to implement a unitary method. Theory for practice must be refined and tested *in* practice. The further development of a unitary method of social work practice, then, will be based on the efforts of practitioners, students and teachers to apply these ideas.

NOTES AND REFERENCES FOR CHAPTER 15

1 See, for example, June E. Neill *et al.*, 'Reactions to integration', *Social Work Today*, vol. IV, no. 15 (11 January 1973).
2 C. Wright Mills, *The Sociological Imagination* (New York: Oxford University Press, 1959), p. 34.
3 Pincus and Minahan, *Social Work Practice*, pp. 112–13. (Italics added.)
4 ibid., p. 73.
5 Goldstein, *Social Work Practice*, p. 10.
6 Purcell and Specht, 'The House on Sixth Street'.
7 Vickery, 'Specialist: generic: what next?'.

INDEX

Printed in the United States
by Baker & Taylor Publisher Services